Welcome to the Bright

The Winding Path from Survivor to Thrivor

Lisa Febre

Black Rose Writing | Texas

ISBN: 978-1-68513-489-1
PUBLISHED BY BLACK ROSE WRITING
www.blackrosewriting.com

Printed in the United States of America
Suggested Retail Price (SRP) $21.95

Welcome to the Bright is printed in Sabon Lt Std

*As a planet-friendly publisher, Black Rose Writing does its best to eliminate unnecessary waste to reduce paper usage and energy costs, while never compromising the reading experience. As a result, the final word count vs. page count may not meet common expectations.

Praise for

Welcome to the Bright

"*Welcome to the Bright* is a glorious testimony to the choices one remarkable young cancer survivor makes both in struggling to navigate post-cancer recovery, and in reflecting on and finding purpose in the life she's lived so far. With honesty, introspection, and wry humor, Febre shines a light on her year after the first clear scan is received, chronicling the debilitating effects of adjuvant therapy, her struggles to move back into a life she's been denied for so long, and the looming fear that the cancer will return.

With grit, grace, and humor, Febre explores a life in which she has not only surrendered to but embraced change and a new way of being. With faith in herself, hunger for knowledge, and the security of being loved, she sets off on a new journey to find her way back to herself.

Drawing hauntingly beautiful parallels between her own experience and the rhythms of the California wilderness in which she immerses herself, Febre spins a captivating and comforting narrative about the power of the self, community, and love. Turning outward, connecting to the vastness of the natural world, Febre's writing is at its most lyrical, starting off quietly and gently, then swelling to a crescendo of awe before calming to a resolute whisper of self-affirmation. *Welcome to the Bright* is a celebration not only of the life we've lived but of the living we have yet to do."

–Troy Hollan, Award-winning author of "*Clucked*"

Welcome To The Bright is an open and sometimes brutally honest recounting of the author's attempt to return to normal following invasive and ravaging Stage IV colon cancer treatments. It's every cancer survivor's dream to get back to "normal," but all too often, the damage done by the very treatments meant to save a life have changed that life forever in ways that will have lasting and sometimes life-altering side effects. Author Lisa Febre's heartfelt retelling is a wakeup call for all of us who know and love someone who has gone through cancer treatment only to discover that our loved ones continue to struggle with long-lasting physical and psychological effects well after they no longer physically look like a cancer patient. A must read for all!

–Barbara A. Luker, Author of " *The Right One*"

"In *Welcome to the Bright,* Lisa continues her symbiotic and spiritual relationships with flora and fauna as she did in *Round the Twist*–the metaphors continuing as a comforting through line.

Reengaging with friends and family after the trauma of cancer, she learned when to lean on her loved ones and caregivers, while always feeling the comforting embrace of Mother Nature. Lisa challenges readers to understand what it feels like to summon the unfair amount of strength necessary to conquer the anxiety she felt in her post-disease universe. *Welcome to the Bright* makes sense of common and complex emotions. "Be it bad or good," we're gifted permission to feel them. Like a park ranger, Lisa has mapped out her journey to bury PTSD into fertile ground and nurture its growth into something as resilient as the manzanita trees she admires during her hikes."

–Traci Asher, Author of " *1 Cancer Patient*"

"With humor and heart, Lisa Febre shares her struggle to regain a new normal as she transitions from cancer patient to cancer survivor. This brave memoir addresses the less-discussed aspects of cancer recovery, including female sexual dysfunction, hair

regrowth, the emotional challenges of weight gain, and the lurking fear that remission could be transient. Febre's eloquent narrative draws parallels between her own journey and the fate of the Miranda Trail she so loves to hike. A truly empowering read that reminds us to care for our loved ones long after the visible challenges of disease have faded."
–Niamh McAnally, Award nominated author of *"Flares Up"*

Lisa Febre's sequel to *Round the Twist* invites the reader into a cancer survivor's viewpoint of her new world, which varies from joyful to cautious to angry to heartbreaking. Again, I learned so much about the effects of cancer, not only on the person themselves but also the people around them, things I never imagined. Skillfully written, the author opens her heart and soul to share her experience with a disease that ravaged her body and spirit, and changed her perspective on life, relationships, and daring to hope.
–AJ McCarthy, Award-winning author of the *"Charlie & Simm"* series

After Survival Comes Healing. Lisa Febre once again shares her heart, her soul, and her journey in this latest look at her life following a diagnosis of colon cancer. And she does it with brutal honesty and her expressive, yet poignant parallels. Her way of comparing the natural world to the human body first amazed me in *Round the Twist* and now does it again in this book.

The first step after a cancer diagnosis is surviving. What one does not often think about is the second step: healing. Ms. Febre's latest work reminds us how while neither is easy, both are necessary in the process of not only surviving cancer but thriving in its frightening aftermath. We often feel that the aftermath of surviving a cancer diagnosis is smooth sailing. But *Welcome to the Bright* helps us to understand that survival is part of a whole new journey.
–Yvonne deSousa, author of *"Shelter of the Monument"*

To Vicky: May your light forever shine bright.

This story chronicles the year between my chemotherapy treatments for metastatic colon cancer. The revelations and experiences I write about within these pages are my own; other survivors may or may not find similarities to their own stories. I am not an expert on colon cancer, but I am an expert on my journey. I hope my words bring some comfort to those who read. I have changed a few of the names for privacy and moved some events around in time for narrative purposes, but everything included in this story happened.

Welcome to the Bright

Part 1

"Lisa, you are meant to be here; you have so much more to do."
–Niamh McAnally

Miranda

Without warning, Luna stopped in her tracks. Lost in my reverie, I almost stepped on her. Most days, I rarely look up to enjoy the scenery because I spend most of our hiking time scanning the trail ahead of Luna for snakes. She is a jumpy dog, not interested in excitement or new things. Like coyotes, she does not approve of changes in her environment. The Miranda Trail is a world of familiar fun things for her. Luna knows the trail better than I do, and today, she was the one who alerted me to the change. A *big* change.

Three months had passed since the world shut down against an invisible enemy: COVID-19. The economy ground to a screeching halt while people quarantined inside their homes. Bickering broke out over the politics of wearing masks, our government officials threw temper tantrums on television, and leadership failed. Restaurants delivered food, office employees worked remotely, and students took classes online. But all of us in the arts community were out of work.

Shortly after moving into our new house, I became so enamored with the park at our doorstep that I trained to become a California State Parks Volunteer. I spent a long day in seminars learning about the Santa Susana Pass State Historic Park from the Park Ranger in charge. We learned to identify various snakes and lizards. Archeologists spoke about the history of the area and their mission to preserve this land with its hidden Native American artifacts. When it was over, I received a name tag and a fancy California State Parks Volunteer patch. With that, I officially became the nerdiest person I knew.

At the beginning of the pandemic, no one fully understood how infectious the virus was; we were told to stay 6-feet apart from everyone in public places. Nervous neighbors crossed the street, afraid to pass too close on the sidewalks. The State Park was closed to the public. I missed my daily hikes, as did the dogs, who were becoming antsy. I checked my email every morning for notices from the State Parks Department, hoping for any news regarding the reopening of the trails. Finally, I got my wish: the park would reopen in the first week of July.

Like a starting gun had gone off, I wasted no time getting back out there. I pulled on my hiking clothes, threw the dogs into their doggie backpacks, and stuffed everyone in the car for the short drive to the park entrance. Hardly able to contain our excitement, we were practically running when I clipped their leashes onto my belt. Finally, we were back on our familiar and much missed trails.

Dusty pranced along next to me, looking up with what I interpreted as a dog smile; Luna rushed ahead of me, pulling her leash into a taut umbilical between us. There was no other option: Luna was leading us straight to the Miranda Trail. It is a one-mile loop up into the hills named after the Francisco Miranda family—homesteaders who staked their claim here in the 1880s. For a while, this land was owned by Roy Rogers and Dale Evans, and the red barn where Trigger lived is walking distance from our house. Now the hills belong to the State Parks Department, and the original Miranda Homestead is used as a cemetery—the tiny adobe house still stands on the property. Often, I venture into the cemetery grounds to jog on the winding paths, enjoying the quiet and lack of traffic.

The Miranda trail has everything the dogs need for a fun morning in the great outdoors: mud, bugs, lizards, rocks to climb on, and coyote poop to sniff. Their quick pace up the hills means

I either must pull them back to slow them down, or just give in and trot behind them. They are the best training partners for trail races.

Usually as we approach the trail, I say to the dogs, "Let's go see Miranda!" As if *Miranda* is a friend who lives on the mountain. The park was open again, but after three spring months with no foot traffic, the trail was overgrown with wildflowers, weeds, and our least favorite stinging nettles. Those scratchy plants would not keep us from enjoying our beloved hike. And in record time, we reached the top, the mid-point of the loop, Luna in the lead, me in the middle, and Dusty prancing up the rear.

That was when Luna came to a screeching halt. There was no question what had upset her. Something terrible had happened here: the chaparral was gone, and pulverized boulders were tossed haphazardly around the edges of the area. The manzanitas had been clear cut, the perfectly sliced, short stumps sticking out of the ground, the corpses of the desert trees left in crude piles. A pair of mourning doves frantically called and hopped between the cut branches, ignoring me and the dogs. This scene played out in the shadow of a small hill blocking the view from the houses below. It looked like the land had been carved by a rabid mountain troll.

The dogs and I stood staring at this destruction, all three of us wary about moving forward and walking through this painful wound on *Miranda's* side. Would the raw land feel our feet and shiver at our touch? We would have to move forward to see just how bad this was.

Our Park Ranger would need to know about this. I dug my phone out of my backpack and snapped several pictures. The dogs waited patiently, as if they understood the seriousness of the situation. *Mom can fix it,* their faith in me unwavering. I just needed faith in myself to follow through with the complicated bureaucratic cure.

Luna and I decided it was out of our hands. We should continue our hike and hope for some justice for our beloved park. Moving across the scar, we discovered some hidden construction equipment behind another mound of boulders. In their shortsightedness to hide their handiwork from view of the houses, the offender overlooked the hiking trail that ran right through the construction site. Hikers were bound to notice the damage sooner or later. My anger was bubbling at the audacity of someone thinking they could just clear land that did not belong to them. The park is not separated from the surrounding area by fences or barbed wire; it is wild, and open. The Parks Department trusted it was safe to leave it the way it was.

The injustice of the whole situation had me worked up for days. My husband, Louis, went back to snap more pictures, this time with Lat-Long coordinates for the archeologists. A map of the State Land superimposed over his photos confirmed this was illegal construction within the park. The State Parks Law Enforcement Department got involved, and the guilty party slapped with a hefty fine, bringing the construction to a halt. Although we had all done our best to save her, our friend *Miranda* suffered severe damage, and she would have to recover from this on her own.

My heart ached. How many birds and animals lost their homes? Without roots and chaparral, could the land withstand even a light rain? I had been a part of the solution. That had to be good enough.

A few months later, a wildfire burned through another two and a half acres of the park. Several helicopters dumped water from above while dozens of firefighters fought flames on the ground. Residents of our neighborhood emptied onto the sidewalks to watch the drama unfold as the giant plume of black smoke rose into the sky. When it was over, the land was bare, burnt, and smelled of fire. Now the park had two wounds: one natural, one artificial.

Within three months of the fire, tiny, deep green buds began poking out from the ashes. Six months later, a carpet of healthy green growth covered the area. The burnt manzanitas stood like blackened skeletons, with fresh shoots reaching up from the ground around their feet. New flames of yellow and purple wildflowers were growing as far as the eye could see. The colors stood in glorious contrast to the brown and black of the surrounding burn area, obscuring the charred boulders. Nature was flourishing after the fire, stronger and even more beautiful than before.

The Miranda clear-cutting was barren and sickly in contrast to the wildfire acres. The manzanita stumps were not sending up shoots. Even common weeds were struggling to get a foothold. This was a serious injury and *Miranda* would need a meaningful amount of time to heal.

Cancer was not a wildfire inside of me. I was not regrowing beautiful wildflowers and lush green succulents on top of fresh tissue. An invading conqueror methodically mowed down my insides and then tried to hide out from the doctors around my body. Cancer was the greedy parasite, devouring my insides and leaving me scarred and damaged. While I hoped I would recover and return to my old self, clearly it would not be that simple. I was damaged, physically and emotionally, and, like *Miranda*, I would also be required to devote a meaningful amount of time and energy to my recovery.

Only two short years later, I was dragging myself along the Miranda Trail with the hope of staying healthy and sane during chemo. I would always stop to stand in this lingering injury. We had so much in common, *Miranda* and me. A hurt that was trying desperately to heal itself. We were two otherwise healthy mountains, with festering wounds on our sides. We could recover together, one tiny weed at a time.

So Many Dreams

When we survive cancer, win the metaphorical battle, and receive that cherished clean bill of health, the expectation is that we instantaneously move on with our lives as if nothing ever happened. The fever has broken; time to get out of bed and back to work. Just like recovering from the flu, the same expectation exists with cancer. We feel better now, which means we are supposed to go back to life exactly as it was before. While I was in treatments, I also believed this would happen when I emerged on the other side of cancer. Having lived it, I know it does not work that way. There is no going back to the way I was or the life I knew. My perspective has changed in ways I may never want to remedy.

My body is healing, and the scars are fading, but my most basic lizard brain and cells remember what happened in primal detail. Parts of my body are still struggling to recover and forget, while other parts are clinging to the trauma and trying to make sure I hear their pain.

The simple act of stepping out of my front door turns into a monumental undertaking. How can I function in a world where I feel so alone? All around me, there are people out there who understand this. They are other cancer survivors. Drawn together, we find comfort and reassurance in knowing that we are not alone in these feelings of isolation from the people around us.

Since my diagnosis, something has inexplicably drawn me to the breeze through the trees. I have spent a lot of time trying to figure out why I now find the trees in our backyard so hypnotic. I stare at the leaves outside the window of my yoga-slash-music room. Even when they are unmoving, they radiate energy and life. I cannot tear my eyes away. After talking to many other cancer survivors, I discovered that *leaves* are a common thread in our post-cancer world. Perhaps we feel the powerful sentience of trees more keenly now. Perhaps a new leaf grows when someone dies. Our energy turned back to the Earth, our life force absorbed by those ancient beings around us with the bark and shivering branches.

I have stood face to face with Death. His eyes fixed intently on my face, with no malice or greed, to offer me a warm invitation. "You don't need to fight this," he whispered, extending a kind hand. "Why put yourself and everyone you love through this ordeal? Just come with me," he beckoned. Calmly, I reached for his hand; he waited patiently as I pondered my answer.

"I'm not ready yet," I decided, my fingertips hovering just out of his reach.

Like an old friend, he tipped his head with a warm smile, and promised, "I'll be here whenever you need me." My heart ached a little as he dissolved into the bright lights of the hospital ceiling.

In December 2021, a surgeon took one look at me and my scans and rushed me into emergency surgery for a bowel blockage. Up to that point, another set of doctors had been dragging their feet to diagnose the underlying problem. In the meantime, my symptoms were getting worse, in particular severe abdominal pain and constipation. It was my new surgeon, Dr. Quilici, who sprung to action the moment he met me, wasting no time in getting me to surgery. I awakened to the news of a Stage-4C colon cancer diagnosis, and a bleak prognosis. During that surgery, I dreamed through the anesthesia. They say it's impossible, but I know I did. I awoke with a jumble of confusing and vibrant images in my head, diluted with morphine. Grasping desperately at what I had seen, I knew I would never remember what had happened to me while I was out. The only thing I could to do to record this experience was to whisper to Louis, "I had so many dreams…"

He thought I meant I had given up; that I knew how bad things were, and I was bemoaning my fate—I may never see my life's ambitions come to fruition. He was understandably upset. But the lines on my forehead were gone; he described my face as child-like, buried in the blankets. It was then that he knew I was speaking literally, not metaphorically.

I may never tap into those anesthesia visions, though I will always hope for a tiny glimpse of the vast universe I traveled. Perhaps it is more important just to know I dreamt than to know what the dreams were.

Back at home, I had four weeks to recover from surgery before chemotherapy started. During that time, I had many dreams—or rather, visions—that brought me immense amounts of comfort and courage. The most important and striking recurring vision was of a dark coven—five figures congregated around my bed. With their disembodied voices, they took it in turns to speak messages meant to help me face down my fears before treatments began. Ahead of my first meeting with my oncologist, Dr. Jacobs, one whispered, "Like a demon needs to give up its name in order to be exorcised, the cancer needs to give up its name in order to be destroyed." "This is all," one told me, encircling Louis and me within a shimmering blue flame. Another showed me a dissolving cancer cell, and said, "Accept chemotherapy into your body as your friend and ally, and you will be healed." During chemotherapy, the fourth gave me the gift of a physical messenger and the reassurance that I had the strength to get through the remaining doses. They have all spoken to me, except for one—and not for lack of trying. Several times she has attempted to make contact, but I have not yet been brave enough to hear her message. Her attempts have frightened me, sending me into full out fear filled with fits and screams.

Trying to hold on to my courage, the thing that would keep me sane and strong during treatments, I grasped on to the important words my oncologist spoke to me at my darkest hour: "This is all temporary." His words helped keep my mind focused on getting through this battle with cancer and finding myself healthy on the other side. "Next year, this will all be a memory," I told myself. I was looking forward to that time in the future and expected I would breathe a tremendous sigh of relief. Instead, when that moment came, I did not have the dramatic relief I thought I would.

"Why is it so hard to accept what you're saying?" I asked Dr. Jacobs. He stood patiently beside my hospital bed, holding my hand, the shepherd in my world of chaos. I was numb, in disbelief, and unable to wrap my brain around the concept of wellness—the thing I had been looking forward to after so many months of fear and uncertainty.

"It takes time to understand this," he said, giving my hand a warm squeeze. "Don't worry, we'll get you there."

In the ten months leading up to this conversation, I fought for my survival with 12 weeks of chemotherapy, 29 radiation treatments, four surgeries, and a colostomy. My life revolved around doctors' appointments, scans, and blood tests, making my pill dispenser the most reliable indicator of the day of the week. Despite all my positivity, optimism, and hope, I could not accept the reality of this moment when he said, "No visible sign of disease." This was a bit more precarious than what we see in the movies when the doctor declares the patient unequivocally cured, and in the next scene, life is magically back to normal. But what I heard was that there was a possibility of invisible disease and that my life was going to be anything but normal again.

It would have been easy to be overwhelmed with resentment and anger by what happened to me. And yet, the memories I had of this period were only positive ones. I thought of the amazing people I met thanks to this stupid disease. Friendships became deeper as I learned I was never alone. As I watched our story unfold in real time, I discovered just how much my husband loved me. With pride, I watched my son take on some very grown-up responsibilities. Cancer opened my eyes to the wonder and beauty of the world all around me. There was more joy than I have ever imagined spilling into every aspect of my life.

I walked out of the hospital after the colostomy reversal surgery, marking the end of the primary treatment of my cancer, under my own power. Cancer had tried to take everything from me. It had stripped away pounds, internal organs, hair, and skin, but it did not strip me of my life.

"Hooray! Hooray! A brand-new day!" resonated in my head. Waking up and opening my eyes is a gift. I promised myself I would chant this mantra with the dogs from now on. Every day deserves a celebration.

The nurse who had accompanied me on this trip back to the outside world was still holding me steady when I stepped through the hospital doors and onto the sidewalk. I may have been weak, but I was determined to make the long walk; I did not want to ride out of the hospital in a wheelchair. After two days in the ward, the bright sun hit my eyes like daggers. I was a newborn baby abruptly thrust into the white light of the world.

Louis, standing by the car, waved, and called out, "Welcome to the Bright!" He rushed over to collect me. I knew he was talking about the sunlight. But at that moment, it seemed like an appropriate title for the second half of my life.

All the doctors told me I had accomplished the impossible. The heavy burden of the statistics pressed on my chest, no matter how positive I was feeling now. Against the odds, I had walked away from this brush with cancer the same way I had walked in: on my own two feet.

I was not cancer-free—yet. I was standing on a hill overlooking the next half of my life. It would be a long hike through the nettles and weeds down the far side of this mountain. Although the nightmare of this round of cancer treatments was behind me, I was facing down an even greater challenge: resuming normal life.

And that might prove even harder than the battle I fought to save it.

Potential Garbage

I wrote a book! In my wildest dreams, I never once imagined that in my late 40s I would add "published author" to my resume. I love to write. I started doing it when I was a child partly because typing on the keyboard is a lot like playing the piano. Both involve moving your fingers to bring ideas to life. And both allow me to communicate with countless people. As a teenager, I gave fake interviews in the mirror with faceless reporters about my imaginary latest album, my latest movie, my latest famous person thing. In high school, I accepted many Grammys in the shower, conspicuously shaped like Finesse Shampoo bottles. Who knew that my claim to fame would be a cancer memoir?

Publishing a book is not a simple process. Two years passed between when I began writing until the first edition rolled off the presses. Writing the book took well over fifteen months, the publishing process added another nine. I began writing just as the diagnosis was beginning in the fall of 2021. I needed an outlet to explore my thoughts and emotions as I faced an uncertain future. At first, I was writing nothing more than brief journal entries on my iPad: "Today I saw Dr. Kagan; this afternoon I got a call from whatever lab; I feel scared, I feel worried; I feel fine, and I wish they would all stop talking about how I might have cancer because, obviously, I don't have cancer." Continuing like this for several months, I never fully understood just how involved this project would become.

I started by posting these journal entries into a blog which I had started on the CaringBridge hosting site—a place for people with any sort of illness to give updates to friends and family. It was the perfect place to announce, "I have colon cancer," and to give a little backstory when I surprised everyone with the news. It would have been thoughtless to drop the bomb in a Facebook post: "Hey everybody, guess what? I have colon cancer." I used the blog platform to give some context before diving into descriptions of the scary stuff. By doing that, I hooked all my blog readers from the start. Opening myself up with honest and raw entries gave people a reason to care about following along with me on this journey. Or maybe my ego just wanted to have another imaginary interview in the mirror. "Remember that musician with all the shampoo awards? She's just been diagnosed with a terminal disease. Follow along as we report on her progress."

It was an honor that so many people subscribed to the blog. But the responsibility that came with writing about my experience in real-time terrified me. Most people seem to know what chemotherapy and radiation are in the technical sense; everyone is familiar with surgery and diagnostic scans like CTs and MRIs. We all know someone with cancer who has been through these things, and of course the internet is there to provide the rest of the details. But Google cannot explain what goes on inside a patient's mind after cancer turns their life upside down. Unless closely involved, one cannot fully understand the effects of cancer on the patient's life. I made the scary decision that my blog would offer something that so many other cancer writers avoided: transparency.

I wrote about my inner turmoil and emotional experience. The side effects of chemo made for interesting reading. But the revelations I was having under the influence of the drugs were what kept people hooked. Some readers told me they got more out of my blog than anything else they had ever read about cancer. It was terrifying to keep writing like that—I learned the hard way that every experience needed to be shared. At one point, I tried to save some of the emotional horrors for myself, believing I could deal with these in private. Ironically, when I gave myself the privacy I was craving, I felt worse. Blowing off steam and letting out the back pressure through writing became an important key to my mental health.

Louis pointed out I was spending more time writing than doing anything else, including practicing my cello, hitting the yoga mat, or hiking. A few doses into my chemotherapy, he suggested I turn my journals into a book that the two of us could use later to remember the experience. I began by changing my journal format from short daily entries to longer musings, trying out topics on the blog to see how people responded, and then exploring them deeper in my personal writings—the project would turn into the book I expected only me and my husband ever to read.

The book ended with my reversal surgery because I felt the colostomy defined my cancer experience—without the colostomy, that part of the journey was clearly over. It was also an uplifting place to stop with my doctors saying they saw "no visible sign of disease." The thing was, I had not stopped writing, and my doctors had not stopped treatments. I was still a cancer patient.

I never imagined that anyone would want to publish any book I wrote. With the encouragement of a longtime friend who is a writer, I prepared a draft of the manuscript for his publisher. When I submitted my manuscript to *Black Rose Writing*, I thought, "This is fun, but it's never going to happen." After hitting send, I went about my business and tried to forget about it. I would self-publish if I needed to, tapping into the knowledge and help of friends who have gone that route before. My Plan B was solid.

Two weeks later, buried between the 45 emails I was mindlessly deleting from my inbox one morning, was a subject line that simply read, "Contract Offer."

Wait. *What?* What kind of contract? I opened the email, and sure enough, *Black Rose Writing* was offering me a book deal. Me! The first publisher to which I submitted my first manuscript was offering me a contract. I shut off my phone, fed the dogs, and stood at the back door, staring out distractedly while they did their post-breakfast business. If the message was still there when I opened my email again, I would know it was real or just my imagination. The dogs came bounding back into the house, tracking little muddy paw prints through my kitchen, but I did not care. I closed the back door, sat down on one of our barstools, and opened the email app again.

"Contract Offer." It was now at the top of the list since I had deleted everything else. But it was still there!

Louis, scuffing in his slippers, appeared from around the corner while I was still staring at my phone screen. He dumped beans in the grinder for our morning coffee, suspiciously eyeing my unusual position at the island. "Why are you sitting there?" He measured my nonresponse. "You look weird."

"I think"—I paused—"this is a contract from that publishing company." Without his reading glasses, he squinted at the email over my shoulder. The teakettle started whistling. Louis turned the flame down and poured the boiling water into the French press. When the kitchen was silent again, I read the message out loud. "It says, 'Lisa, we feel strongly that your project will make a successful addition to our publishing house. I am excited about adding an author with such high potential to the Black Rose Writing Family.'"

"Hear that," Louis smiled. "An author with high potential!" He kissed my cheek as he set a mug down in front of me. "I have always known you were a talented writer."

I just kept shaking my head and repeating, "Who would want to read this?"

He laughed warmly. "You'll see," he said. "This is going to be important."

I may not have known what getting a book into print would entail, but I knew it was about to overtake my life. Thankfully, I could do it all from the safety and comfort of home. I could continue to work on deepening the ass-print on the patio sofa cushion while I did the early proofreading on the same iPad I had written the book. There would be no phone calls or in-person meetings to attend. I had an official excuse to turn down social invitations because, "I'm just so swamped with working on the book." Of course, my favorite one made me feel like an actual writer: "I have a deadline to meet."

After signing the contract, I went to work taking care of all the elements that the publisher needed. First, I would have to finish the manuscript. I also needed to scour my contacts list for published writers to review drafts of the book. For the next month, I tidied up the manuscript into a form I felt comfortable sending out and was blown away when they wrote official sounding reviews; I cried when I read each one of them. One author sent in her review with the comment, "I can't wait to read part two. I hope you're working on it already!"

Until she brought it up, I had not even thought about another book, even though I already had another 20,000 words beyond the end of *Round the Twist*. I was 25% of the way into a sequel, regardless of if I had planned it that way. Taking her request to heart, I collected all the extra chapters all into a new project file and promptly forgot about it. Approaching it the same way I did the first book, I would write when I felt like it, and always with the assumption that it was complete garbage. "Just get it down, and don't worry about if *you* think it's any good," she advised me when I told her I was taking her suggestion seriously.

I struggled mightily with my mental state during the editing process of *Round the Twist*. It was difficult to read and reread the book dozens of times over the following six months. Someone famously said you need to read your manuscript so many times that you become sick of it, and I was well past that point. It was making me emotionally and physically sick. Knowing something horrible was about to happen on the next page, a sense of impending dread would come over me. I had to shut off the computer and get away from the words. Usually, I went to the patio to stare at the trees in the backyard. Sitting in the ridiculously oversized rocking chair (a hilarious purchase Louis made without reading the dimensions in the catalogue), my feet sticking straight out over the seat like the classic Lily Tomlin skit, helped lighten my mood. The dogs would come to me, staring up at me with their big brown eyes, knowing something was wrong and hoping their mere presence could fix me. I hoped my reaction to the book was just because I'd had to relive the worst year of my life so many times, and this was not the effect it would have on the people who bought it. I wanted readers to feel something, but I did not want them to feel sick.

My professional musical life was not all that I had hoped it would be. No matter how I tried to sugarcoat it or convince myself that I was doing something worthwhile, I was always frustrated. Even before cancer, I knew I had not accomplished nearly half of what I had set out to do after college. I was not playing with a professional symphony orchestra, nor teaching at a university. I did not pursue a master's or doctorate degree. When I moved to Los Angeles in 2010, I had aspired to play in the recording studio orchestras—I had only done that a few times, and clearly, that would be it unless my Fairy Godmother finally showed up. My music career never quite got a solid foothold in Los Angeles. Most of what I was doing at that point was for free or for very little money. Not that I got into music to make money, but I do not think it unreasonable to expect a living wage for my life's passion.

Never mistake an intelligent person for someone who enjoys school. As a child, the school placed me into a program for gifted children. I have a near photographic memory, which meant I never had to study. Ever. I graduated college Magna Cum Laude, having barely cracked open a single book—during my junior and senior years, I never even bought textbooks; instead, I pocketed the book money my parents sent me. I could have been anything I wanted. My mother dreamed I would be a doctor. My father probably had plans for me to be an engineer like him, considering how much I loved to take apart watches and electronics; my oboe teacher suggested I become an instrument repair technician because I loved to tinker with all my musical instruments. All I knew was that I wanted to be a musician. In all these years, I came close. But not quite.

In fact, I never had a stable music career which I could settle into for the long haul. For the first fifteen years after college, I restarted my career three times when I moved to three new states. No wonder I could never get past the predictable early stages and land a permanent job. When I met Louis and moved to Los Angeles, I was 35. Career reset number four. I was losing interest and enthusiasm by this point. Perhaps I would have to resign myself to a life without accomplishments. Depression over my career had been my constant companion for years. Thankfully, Louis was expert at recognizing the symptoms each time they reared their ugly heads and supported me through the bumps in the emotional road. Besides using me on most of his own projects, he pulled whatever strings he could to get me some studio work now and then.

Amazing things were happening now. I worked on book two and tried to get back to living my life. I watched the words appear on the screen as if I were an observer, not the writer. And I was learning about myself with each new paragraph, each new idea, each new topic. I tried to face down the thoughts and feelings that I had not tackled because I had been too busy trying to survive cancer. As I got to know myself from a new perspective, I learned I was not the Character Lisa I was an expert at presenting to the world. I was Actual Lisa, a complicated, delicate, and surefooted creature.

Cancer gave me the opportunity to reassess my life honestly and objectively as an outside observer. Would I pick up my music career where I left off and just plow ahead like a stubborn ox? Or was this the time to try something different? This writing thing was working out pretty well. Maybe I should pursue this. I was being asked to write articles for the United Ostomy Association of America (UOAA) website, and I was publishing a steady stream of blogs on my personal webpage. My brain was always planning the next chapter or the next anecdote I would write about. I rushed to the computer every morning to type about whatever thoughts were bouncing around inside my head all night.

Between spurts of writing inspiration, I threw myself into the publicity and marketing needed for *Round the Twist*. Speaking with other cancer survivors made me realize I was a part of something bigger than myself. My new path was not paved in praise and accolades for a book. It was about using writing as the tool through which I give freely of myself and connect with other people. Going into this next period of my life, I had a lot to think about. And luckily, I had a lot of time in which to do that.

I fought hard for my life and sanity. With late-stage colon cancer, I knew things were bad. It would not be an easy road to recovery. But I never once thought that I might actually die. Despair or hopelessness did not cloud my mind, because I simply believed a full recovery waited at the end of this thing. Now that I was on the other side, it was time to decide what to do with the second half of my life, and I needed to approach that process the same way I confronted cancer.

Fear was never in control of my journey. I was.

Cancerversary

I was crying again.

To fully experience whatever it was I was feeling, and not fight it, was a skill I had been expertly honing over the last year. It was naïve to assume that just because the surgeon had said he saw no visible sign of disease, I would spring back upright and miraculously become emotionally stable again.

Today was December 9, 2022. On this date exactly one year ago, I received the unbelievable diagnosis of Stage-4C Colon Cancer at 47. My life was instantly turned upside down. Dealing with the physical side of treating cancer was the simple part. It was the emotional and mental journey that took the most energy and effort. The body recovered, the incisions closed, and the systems regulated. But the wounds in my head felt like they would never heal. I am openly proud of the map of red incisions on my abdomen, but I am terrified to examine the complex spider web of thin silver scars crisscrossing my soul.

The pressure building in my chest forced me to stop in the middle of my yoga practice. I already knew from the past year that just because I felt something, it did not mean I had to name it. It was ok to feel whatever I felt. I had to learn to accept that there might not be a label to attach to every emotion. This day was no different. As far as yoga goes, I was doing a pretty simple thing—lying on my back and hugging my knees into my chest to help my lower back recover from the difficult pose I had just performed. So there was no reason for my heart to be pounding so hard still. Taking a deep breath was becoming difficult, so I let go of my legs and laid there flat on my back like a corpse, waiting for the tightness in my chest to subside so I could think straight.

I stared at the lamp hanging from the ceiling and wondered when that one light bulb had gone out. Everything is supposed to be perfect in my yoga-slash-music room because this is my sanctuary, my safe space for exploring yoga, playing my cello, and working on my book. There is not supposed to be a light bulb out, or a ball of dog hair tumbling across my freshly swept floor, or the brumming of a chainsaw drifting in through my window from somewhere in the neighborhood.

The clove oil I had added to my diffuser was hitting me in the most pleasant way, triggering memories of when my son Andrew was a toddler. Back in New England, stuck indoors on snowy winter days, we would poke cloves into oranges, making our hands and the house smell cozy and delicious. Maybe if I could relax and hold on to this memory, I could hold off the tears and get back to the present moment.

I ran through my now-routine mental checklist: "Are you injured?" *No.*

"Are you sick?" *No.*

"Are you in pain?" *No.*

"Then what's the problem?"

It might be cancer, the voice whispered back.

Right now, everything was ok. I was ok. As far as everyone was concerned, I was not fighting any active cancer. No matter how cognizant I was of that simple fact, the tears continued to leak from my eyes. I brushed them aside, annoyed at myself for this rush of emotion that had come on for no apparent reason. As we move through the familiar sequence of poses, yoga can dredge up deeply embedded feelings and force us to identify, experience, and then release them. It has happened to me before, so there was comfort in knowing this was not anything strange or unexpected. In a few minutes, the feelings would pass, and I would resume my practice. Still, I was annoyed.

Breathe in through my nose—I can ask Louis to replace the lightbulb later; and out through my mouth—I can sweep up the dog hair when I finish yoga. Slowly breathe in again—the chainsaw will eventually run out of gas; and then blow it all away through my mouth—I am doing ok.

I needed to embrace, not erase, the emotion. As I slowly relaxed, the uninvited, as-of-yet unnamed emotion continued to circulate through my body, pure energy.

What am I so angry about? It surprised me when the words entered my mind so easily. But there it was: I was angry. I had reached a point where I was sitting with the emotion and allowing it to speak to me in its own unclouded voice.

This time, I had the experience of a full year behind me, giving me the ability to recognize this simple emotion I was feeling. Plain old anger. A familiar friend I could sit with. Anger often covered me like a blanket made of monster fur, while I sipped a cup of fuming hot cocoa buried under furious little marshmallows.

Now that I had named the emotion, the real fun could begin.

I was angry. And I was also sad and lost, even though I was feeling joyful and victorious sometimes. Overall, I enjoyed a charmed life—a theory which had never been tested quite as strenuously as it had with cancer.

Someone else, standing over my angry little self lying there on the yoga mat, would have seen something quite miraculous. Exactly one year ago, on this day, the doctors had given me a slim chance of surviving one year—they expected me to be dead by now. I never fully appreciated the sentiment until long after the major battles were behind me. Things were bad. But I did not know it had been *not-likely-to-live-out-the-year* bad. It was very lonely being the person who had to come to terms with that prognosis, long after the excitement of the actual battle had passed, and the audience had left the theater. Hindsight reveals things to be more frightening in retrospect than when they were actually happening.

Despite everything that had happened to me, I could still do most of the same advanced yoga poses I did before cancer. There was so much to celebrate. Yet here I was marinating in an angry brine. What was I so angry about? I only knew that I was feeling it. *It's ok to be angry*, I reassured myself. *Who wouldn't be?*

I had always taken care of my body with my decades long, well-established daily fitness routine alternating between Ashtanga yoga and trail running in the hills. I was always moving, always trying to get stronger, and always setting goals for my body. I have every right to be angry that fitness did not spare me from cancer.

I went vegetarian when I was 16, ultimately going vegan when I was 30—a lifestyle to which I have been devoted for two-thirds of my life. There are plenty of studies out there proclaiming that vegans are supposed to be at a much lower risk for colon cancer in particular. JAMA Internal Medicine Journal proclaims that a pescatarian diet (dominated by fruits, vegetables, and a moderate amount of fish) is associated with a reduced risk for colorectal cancers compared to people who eat meat[1]. They also concluded that vegans have an even lower risk compared to vegetarians. We are supposed to be safer than everyone else. In the social media vegan-community groups to which I belong, the spectrum of conversation runs from the rational presentation of the above research to the most outlandish claims that veganism not only prevents but *cures* cancer. I have turned into an obnoxious spoil sport who comes along to contradict all the commenters. My mission has become to point out this utter rubbish, and to suggest that instead of wasting time sharing useless articles about how crushing garlic

---

[1] https://health.clevelandclinic.org/the-best-diet-to-lower-your-colon-cancer-risk-2/

versus chopping it is the cure for colon cancer, they should spend it on the phone with their doctor to schedule a colonoscopy. I am angry that I have to shout into the headwinds of disinformation.

Of the four chemotherapy drugs in my regimen, one of them, Oxaliplatin, left me with lingering neuropathy. Nine months after chemotherapy ended, my fingers still prickled when I played my cello and the pinky toes on both of my feet were numb. Without shoes, I was tripping while walking around the house and often I cut my toenails so short that the quick would bleed. The cold sensitivity in my hands and feet continued as well. Walking around barefoot on the cold hardwood floors was still out of the question. After showers, I hopped from bathmat to bathmat because the floor tiles were too cold. I was still dropping silverware and unable to hold drinks with ice. I was angry that the side effect was lasting so long. But I came to accept that it may be with me for years.

By the time I had broken down in tears on my yoga mat, three months had passed since my colostomy reversal surgery, and I had been on the adjuvant chemotherapy pill for the last two. The first wave of side effects had been so dramatic that Dr. Jacobs reduced the dosage with each round. We would have to find a level that I could tolerate if I were to stay on the drug long-term. I was angry that the pill might not end up being the easy maintenance therapy it promised to be. If the new lower dose did not work for me, I might have to go back on the 5FU. Never in my life had I been someone who routinely took medications. I had every right to be angry that my blood was now a pharmaceutical slurry.

Although I found all this annoying, there was nothing so terrible going on. I decided I could live with all of it—the most important word in that sentence being *live*.

The wave of anger and tears was ebbing. I listened to the soft music that was playing through my speaker, imagining I was floating on those chords like a piece of driftwood in the middle of the sea. Comforted by the calm imagery, I realized I was not lost in a vast ocean. I was exactly where I was supposed to be. And where I was was pretty darn amazing.

During chemotherapy and radiation, I was just lucid enough to rationalize what was happening. The drugs helped me close off parts of my consciousness, so I perfected the skill of distancing myself from the reality of it all. It was the only way I could cope with the outrageous circumstances. Louis was the one who had to watch anxiously as I lost weight, my skin peeled off, and my face contorted from the muscle spasms. Focused on surviving cancer and enduring the drugs, I was not concerned with what the side effects looked like to everyone.

Dr Jacobs had flat out laughed at me at a recent appointment when I claimed that my FOLFIRINOX chemotherapy "wasn't that bad." He shook his head with exasperation. "Oh Lisa," he threw up his hands. "You didn't see what we saw."

I never really thought about it that way until the ordeal was over. Although my spotty recollection portrayed me as having been ok, when Louis and I compared notes, his sober version of events betrayed my memories. It left me reeling at how completely the drugs had wiped out my memory, allowing my mind to protect itself from what was happening to me. Perhaps it appears delusional now, because I spent most of the weeks on chemotherapy struggling and suffering, but in my head, I always felt strong and optimistic. Never once did I think, "I can't survive this." I have my brain to thank for this small kindness.

The odds were stacked against me. Cancer had consumed over six inches of my sigmoid colon, blew up my left ovary to the size of a grapefruit, spread to six lymph nodes, and crept onto the peritoneal wall. The scariest part was the cancer had already metastasized to my liver by the time I had a concrete diagnosis. No matter how I tried to color what was going on, those liver tumors were definitive proof of metastasis. No more denying what was happening to me. Those tumors were as clear as could be on the scans—they forced me to accept that something was seriously wrong. After surgery, the pathologist had his turn, and when the numbers were added up, my cancer staging was 4C (pT4a pN2a pM1c). The end of the line.

And yet, two weeks later, I was back on the yoga mat and hitting the hiking trails. Despite being a little more tired than usual, it was almost as if nothing had even happened. I was learning to live with the colostomy and trying to gain some weight—I had lost 16 pounds. But I was strong and physically ready to face the six doses of chemotherapy that sat patiently waiting for me on the horizon.

In May 2022, seven weeks after chemotherapy ended, I was back on the operating table undergoing an exploratory surgery. One month later, Intensity Modulated Radiation Therapy (IMRT) blasted my body to eradicate the last remaining small cancerous implants—the tiny metastatic tumors from the original cancer which the chemotherapy had left behind. Radiation proved even more difficult on my body than chemotherapy, draining me of strength with unrelenting diarrhea, abdominal pain, and dangerously low blood pressure. I needed to have IV hydration before each of the last six treatments, just to make it through in one piece. Although I had moments of despair, I still showed up at the office day after day until the regimen was complete.

I was exceptionally lucky that the radiation did its job. In September, ten months after my diagnosis, a clear PET showed no remnants of the cancer, and even promised a successful reversal surgery. During that surgery, Dr. Quilici took an extensive look around inside me, reversed my colostomy, and declared there was "no visible disease present."

It was time to get back to real life, reconnect with friends, and maybe even get back on stage. I was looking forward to packing my cello in the Subaru and taking on some winter holiday concerts. The possibilities were endless. Compared to surviving cancer, I expected everything that came next would be a piece of cake.

I pulled my knees back up to my chest, picking up where I had left off in my practice. I rocked slowly side to side like a baby, massaging my stiff lower back, then rolled to my side, and gently pushed myself up to a sitting position. Sitting quietly, I contemplated my next move: would I continue to follow the Ashtanga Series I had been practicing, or would I veer off course? My body told me I needed to do poses that spoke to me at that moment. I felt like flipping upside down for some headstands.

My view of my yoga-slash-music room now flipped upside down, I breathed deeply in a comfortable headstand. A yoga teacher had once advised our class, "When life feels out of control, flip yourself upside down and it will all look right again." She knew what she was talking about. From this viewpoint, the only thing I could see were my cellos against the opposite wall. They stood eagerly waiting for me to pick them up again. Since it was impossible to move my head around with the weight of my body resting on it, I could see nothing else. No other distractions. The message was clear: the second half of my life was waiting for me to join in. It was not impatient; it was sitting in a beautiful handmade wooden body with four strings, perfectly in tune, and full of possibilities.

Slime

Having a colostomy was never on my bucket list. Before having mine, I had never heard of this thing. Like me, most people are unaware of how common they are—the United Ostomy Association of America (UOAA) estimates there are at least one million people living with a colostomy in the United States (not counting those with an ileostomy or urostomy). There are people who call it *a bag* with an unadorned air of disgust, which I always find insulting. Everyone poops. People with a colostomy just do it a little differently.

This past year, I read a celebrity memoir in which he recounted the events leading up to his bowel rupture, resulting in him being given a temporary colostomy. There was not a single sympathetic word written about the colostomy; the whole thing was disheartening. His description disappointed me. Hundreds of thousands of people would read his memoir and walk away from it thinking that colostomies are the worst thing that can happen to someone. He leads the reader to believe that a colostomy is disgusting and embarrassing. He had a genuine opportunity to shine a light on this lifesaving procedure—to show the world that if a celebrity can manage one of these, then there is hope for us regular people. Instead, he chose to paint the situation in the opposite light, and I was crushed. Disappointed and deflated, I wrote him a letter. It forever lives in a folder on my computer; I will never send it.

I worked very hard, after awakening with the colostomy, to come to terms with the drastic change inflicted upon my body and mind. Although I was told it was temporary, I doubt anyone had the inside scoop on that one. Given my poor prognosis, the assumption was that I would not live long enough for a reversal. So, why not give me something to hope for? Seemingly past the scary stuff, I felt ready to face this dismal view of the situation. I even felt brave enough to ask Dr. Quilici if my assumption was true.

During the ten months I had my colostomy, I tried to portray it as not a big deal and just another medical condition, hoping I might be an ambassador for the world of Ostomates. I snapped pictures of myself doing yoga with the appliance showing. I went hiking and running, even competing in a 5K race with the bag tucked into my running shorts. I encouraged my friends and family to have a look at it, and many took me up on the offer. Many people told me they learned something about ostomies and felt better equipped to support other people in the future.

Dr. Jacobs was always apologetic about it. Week after week, month after month, he would say, "Don't worry, I'll make sure that it's actually temporary." But I felt a lot of gratitude toward it. The excruciating pain I had endured for months vanished when the surgeon removed the cancerous portion of my colon. The colostomy, though a sad token of that insidious cancer, was also a positive reminder of what it took to stay alive. Missing that stretch of colon, losing all that parasitic cancer, left a gap in my plumbing, and yet I was thriving. I was alive, it was important for me to accept the medical procedure that granted me more time on this planet.

After 12 weeks of chemotherapy, they sent me to surgery to assess just how well it had worked to kill the cancer. I also knew that Dr. Quilici would evaluate the possibility of reversing the colostomy. It all depended on how badly the cancer had damaged my rectum. I made the mistake of mentioning the reversal on my blog. In hindsight, I should have shut up about it and only written about the exploratory portion of the surgery.

Unfortunately, people mainly focused on the reversal. There were a lot of comments expressing relief and excitement that "Your ordeal would soon end." But they were not talking about the cancer itself. I was confused and frustrated, chasing comments on my blog, and answering a tidal wave of emails and texts from people who could not wait for my colostomy to go away. In my mind, *The Ordeal* I was going through was not the colostomy. It was the very serious, late stage, terminal cancer and its treatments which had ravaged every cell in my body. Chemotherapy was more dramatic and damaging to my body than the colostomy. And instead of being able to focus on my excitement at possible good news regarding the cancer, I was feeling defensive about my colostomy.

When I awoke from the surgery with the colostomy still in place, I felt vindicated. *What now, people? What do you have to say about this?* I hit the blog, almost daring people to cross me. I would not apologize or soothe other people's feelings on the matter. Instead, I enjoyed watching them twist and squirm to convince me it was alright to still have the colostomy. The Grinch in me loved watching them try to convince themselves under the guise of soothing me.

Radiation treatments took up much of that summer. I had a severe reaction to IMRT; all my doctors tried desperately to keep me out of the hospital by giving me daily intravenous hydration until it was over. Until this point, I had been on the drug Xeloda (Capecitabine). Combined with the dehydration, the drug had contributed to a sudden drop in blood pressure. In an uncharacteristic show of indignation and fanfare, Dr. Jacobs promptly took me off it.

The damage the radiation caused to the organs in my pelvis was severe. I had been told to get back on the yoga mat as soon as possible after treatments ended to prevent scar tissue from limiting the range of motion in my pelvis, hips, and lower back. In the nine weeks between radiation and my next surgery, I focused on being gentle yet persistent while trying to work out the new tightness so I could get back my full range of motion.

Another attempt at a reversal loomed on the horizon. Would it be successful this time? Of course, I hoped so. The emotional rollercoaster leading up to the surgery was a wild ride. I was not counting down the days to the surgery with excitement. In fact, I had quite a bit of anxiety and trepidation. As the days ticked by, my attachment to my stoma was increasing. I was sorry that it would be chopped off and incinerated after all it had done for me. I was sad to see my stoma go. The colostomy satisfied my need to stand out. I welcomed the questions and curiosity, and I enjoyed talking about it both in my support group and amongst my curious friends. It made me feel special, and I could already feel I would miss the attention when it was gone.

This time around, I did not post a single word about the reversal on my blog—I kept calling the surgery "exploratory." I would not put myself through the same public ordeal as the previous surgery. If I had the reversal, I would announce it; if not, then no one would know it had even been on the table. I hoped I was saving myself a lot of grief.

We take for granted how a well-oiled digestive tract works, unseen and unsupervised. We never give our colon a second thought until it makes a strange noise or gives us grief. With a colostomy, there is a closeness and familiarity with your inner workings most people never get to experience. I knew how long it took for my guts to move after I ate a meal, so I knew when to stop eating in the evening to prevent a full bag from waking me during the night. I had direct contact with an internal organ I would have never seen otherwise. The digestive tract fascinated me, and I spent many afternoons reading med school materials online. And, at one appointment, I even declared to Dr. Quilici, that if I were a little younger, I might consider going back to school to become a bariatric surgeon. "What's stopping you?" He was a little more enthusiastic than I would have preferred.

"I'm pretty squeamish, and I really don't want to go back to school," I laughed.

"Well," he nodded along. "You would get over being squeamish quickly. But unfortunately, there is a lot of schooling involved." We settled the matter: I would not be a surgeon in my middle age.

Even without a guaranteed reversal, I still had to go through the bowel prep the night before. Much like what we go through before a colonoscopy, except that there are three rapid doses of heavy antibiotics taken along with it. The colon and bowel are full of bacteria which, if leaked into our abdominal cavity during or after surgery, could cause a deadly infection. It also gives us a fighting chance against any infections popping up after the surgery, sabotaging a successful reversal.

I am not proud to say I cried during the bowel prep that day. There had been a recall of the kinder and gentler magnesium citrate, so the pharmacy gave me that horrible Suprep drink. Two doses of that were hard enough to choke down six hours apart, but the hospital pharmacy had given me the set of antibiotics in suspensions. Unlike my surgery prep in May, when they gave me the antibiotics in tablet form, I had to mix up these concoctions myself.

Just thinking about the antibiotics makes me nauseous. The doses came in segregated bottles: three bottles of powdered antibiotic, three bottles of the suspension liquid. I am being very generous in calling it *liquid*—I took chemistry in high school, and this thick goo was anything but liquid. When we were kids in the 1980s, my brother, Todd, was obsessed with play slime. He would cover his action figures in it, cover his hands in it, and chase me around, claiming that it was neon green boogers. It got in our hair and our bedroom carpets. It had a distinctive smell, like chemicals and plastic. It was disgusting then, and believe me when I say it was just as disgusting trying to drink something like it for my bowel prep. Who on earth thought this was a good idea?

I had to choke down those suspensions every two hours, and by the last one, I was gagging. When Louis found me, I was on our bed crying as waves of nausea crashed over me. He saw me go through chemo and radiation without vomiting. He knew just what to do—he brought out my stash of Zofran, certain that the anti-nausea medication would work just as well as it did during chemo. Thankfully, it did. But if we needed to postpone this surgery into the future, I would have to consider carefully how badly I wanted it. Going through this ordeal again might not be worth it.

I tried to go into the surgery with a positive attitude, but underneath the façade, I was terrified. This was major surgery. The bowel is dangerous territory: chopping it up and sewing it back together again is fraught with risks. Ten years earlier, the father of Andrew's best friend had died after this same surgery. In his late 40s, he too had beaten colon cancer. Only difference was he died from complications from his reversal because the surgeon accidentally nicked his intestine. He succumbed to a massive infection within days.

His story was something I tried hard to suppress in the 24 hours before my surgery. "It did not happen at our hospital," Louis reminded me multiple times that day as I was prepping for surgery. It will not happen to me. I needed to believe I would not die. By now, Louis was expert at soothing this fear, and kept repeating to me, "Dr. Quilici is one of the best surgeons in Los Angeles. He would never make that sort of mistake." I had to trust Louis' confidence was solid enough for me to stand on as well.

The next day, I awoke from surgery with not just a clean bill of health, but also a reconnected colon. Five o'clock in the morning after my surgery, Dr. Jacobs came to my hospital room to tell me that Dr. Quilici had seen no sign of disease in my pelvis. I had three hours between his news and the start of visiting hours when Louis could join me for the day. It was so difficult for me to understand the good news that I decided I would not even think about it until Louis got there. It was possible he would celebrate with me and say, "This is great!" But it seemed more likely he would say, "You're delusional. Dr. Jacobs hasn't even been to see you yet." Louis would confirm this had not been a dream.

I was still struggling with weight loss after radiation. The liquid diet and bowel prep ahead of surgery had robbed me of two more pounds. My entire digestive tract had been emptied—now it was telling me to fill it back up. The nurses viewed my morning hunger as an encouraging sign of quick healing. The only downside was having to spend a few more hours on a liquid diet, putting my dreams of solid food on hold until dinner.

Dr. Quilici caught up to me in the hallway that afternoon while I was working on my required laps; the metal pole of the IV tree had to be wrapped in a towel, since I still had cold sensitivity from the recent chemo. Pleased with what he saw, he said I could go home right away. Any rational person would have jumped at the chance to leave the hospital. Not me. Even though everything seemed to go smoothly with my quick recovery, the memory of our friend destabilized me. What if something terrible happened after I got home? We lived 30 minutes away from the hospital. That would be a long drive with internal bleeding or worsening sepsis.

I had banked a lot of goodwill with this man over the past year. It was time to cash it in. "Is it possible to stay one more night?" I negotiated.

"It's up to you," one corner of his mouth tightening into a sideways grin as he considered my request. "Tomorrow you go home, though," he countered.

"Tomorrow for sure," I agreed. We settled the matter with a tip of our heads instead of a handshake.

One more night under the watchful eyes of my favorite nurses would make me feel much better. Besides, I was so sore from all the incisions. It would be nearly impossible to keep the dogs from jumping on me. How would I move around our house or get in and out of our bed? At the hospital, my IV tree acted as a security blanket. Holding on to it made me feel safe going to the bathroom by myself. I was not ready to let go of it just yet.

The next day, I was feeling so well that I was eager to get home and see my son and my dogs, and to sleep in my bed with my husband next to me. Nothing soothes the soul better than being in your own environment, amongst your family and away from the chaos that a hospital ward injects into your recovery. I took my enthusiasm for returning home as the sign that things were going just fine inside of me.

Also, the hospital was not the place I wanted to experience my first real bowel movements. I was nervous about how my intestines would restart. What mysteries awaited me as they began working on their own? For ten months, my rectum was not attached to anything, which meant my anal muscles had been on an extended vacation. I worried about having accidents as I relearned how to use the toilet. Recovery is highly individual. No one could fully prepare me. This is where my colostomy support group was the most useful, as those who have had reversals shared their stories and laid out the timelines for their return to normal bathroom habits.

I did not know what to expect. I had been passing a lot of gas in the hospital, which was expected given the amount of air that they pumped into my colon and abdomen during the surgery. Each time I farted, I worried incisions were tearing apart. When Louis was around, I would press a finger to my lips and sheepishly bat my newly regrown eyelashes at him. With my ridiculously curly hair growing out of control, the whole scene made us laugh even harder. There was nothing ladylike about the first few days after my surgery. Of course, I would never miss the opportunity to put on a good show.

Sherry, a new friend from the colostomy support group, texted me just after I arrived back home. She had her successful reversal eight weeks before me and was very forthcoming with the details about her recovery. "Don't be scared, but your first bowel movement is going to look like a murder scene." She followed this statement with a line of poop emojis followed by the request, "Don't send pictures!"

When the sensations finally hit me, just a few hours after I returned home, I barely had time to make it to the bathroom. My poor muscles were weaker than I had expected. But I made it, and Sherry was right: it was a frightening sight! It was largely the blood and goo left over from surgery. I felt much better, though.

Walking into the living room like a triumphant Olympian, I stretched my arms into the air and stuck my chest out. "I did it!" I exclaimed.

"Good girl!" Louis laughed as he threw me a high-five. "Do you want a cookie?" We were dying; this could be a lot of fun if we allowed ourselves to enjoy it.

One more urgent trip to the bathroom that evening seemed to clear out what else remained of the surgical leftovers. Between the pain from the surgery and my questionable bowel control, I hoped I could make it through the night. I would need his help to get out of bed if anything happened in the wee hours.

My abdominal muscles were so sore and weak, the new incision made any slight movement a misery. It was still uncomfortable to lie flat on my back, so I was using a foam back support to keep me upright, and a wedge under my knees to spare my lower back. "This is all temporary," I chanted, reminding myself that each day would bring noticeable recovery. Just had to stay patient.

"What if I poop in the bed?" I asked Louis, as he helped me hoist my legs up and covered me with the blankets.

"Then I clean the bed," he said.

"In the middle of the night?" I moaned.

"We still have some puppy pads. Do you want me to put one under you?" he twinkled. But that was too much for me.

"Forget it! I'll just squeeze my butt cheeks as hard as I can!" With this much laughter, pooping the bed might be inevitable.

Potty training resembled what toddlers go through. I would feel the urge to go and literally run to the bathroom. I never had an accident, but I pushed the limits a few times. The first two weeks following the surgery, I had many post-op appointments with various doctors. Operating within tight tolerances, I was never confident that I could make it through the car ride and the appointments without an accident. The longest I could go without using a toilet was about two hours—between our 30-minute car ride combined with the hour it would take to see the doctors, I was cutting it very close. I had to use the knowledge I had gained while I had the colostomy to my advantage now: no eating before the appointments meant no pooping my pants in the waiting room.

Everyone is different with how the recovery and restart progresses. For weeks, I was tied to the bathroom. Sometimes I would start pulling up my pants and suddenly need to go again. The sigmoid colon is the collection chamber, holding the feces until the rectum sends you the message that it may be time to find a toilet. Without the sigmoid colon, I have a shortened path from my descending colon into my rectum. Although Dr. Quilici gave me a make-shift sigmoid during surgery, the man-made curve was nowhere near as big as my natural one had been. Sometimes, I was running to the bathroom multiple times per hour. My baby bum was sore, and I used diaper cream to soothe the delicate skin. Was this how my life would be from now on? I wondered if I had made the right choice to have the reversal. The colostomy was a breeze compared to this craziness.

Sherry, lifesaver that she is, reassured me that as the weeks go by, our bodies adjust to their new normal. For her at least, the eight-week mark had been a big milestone. "You'll see," she texted. "Everything will be alright."

She was right. By eight weeks I was visiting the bathroom less and less, and by twelve weeks I was settling into a manageable routine. If, before my colostomy, I used to go to the bathroom twice each day, at three months post-op, I was going eight times. Closing in on the one-year post-reversal milestone, my routine was even more manageable—using the bathroom four times per day. Was that so bad?

The surgery left quite a few scars on my lower abdomen. The stoma closure runs diagonally above my left hip. There is a large, six-inch vertical incision from my pubic bone to just under my belly button, and many poke holes from the laparoscopic portion of the surgery (and all the other surgeries that year) sprinkled around my belly. Because I am fair skinned, I formed keloid cysts over every single incision—they still stood out from my skin, red and angry, one-year post-op. Glimpsing these scars in the mirror, I would boil over with frustration and disgust. What a mess I was. Still very thin, I had all these scars with the tattoo dots from radiation peppered between them. I had to learn how to change my thinking to focus on the positive. Other than my short hair, there was no visible proof I had been through a battle for my life. Except the scars under my clothes.

Louis had a colorful description: "You look like you've been chewed on by an alligator." I agreed. Cancer was the meanest alligator around. I had taken the first round.

Instead of resenting the battle scars, I hoped they would never fade.

(Technically) Disease Free

While I was recovering from the reversal surgery, I had to, of course, announce the results of the exploratory portion of the surgery to my blog readers, friends, family, and anyone else who inquired. With little extra energy to devote to writing, texting, or answering the phone, the sense of responsibility balancing on my shoulders overwhelmed me. I wondered when exactly the tides had shifted, and I became the one required to make everyone else feel better about my situation.

Something I learned during my treatments, or rather at the end of each set of treatments, was that I was profoundly uncomfortable giving everyone a reason to celebrate. I hated the congratulatory emails and was annoyed by any messages that hinted at a celebration. I even became upset watching television shows or movies that portrayed someone receiving an overly dramatic "You're cured!" declaration from their doctor for any condition, be that cancer or the flu. The common expectation is we become Superman in reverse: we walk out of the doctor's office, button up our shirt over our cape, put our glasses back on, and go back to living our lives in anonymity.

I did not celebrate when chemotherapy ended and I refused to cheer when the first surgery found only a little cancer left to treat. I had no interest in celebrating the end of radiation. And now I was actively pushing back when told "no visible sign of disease." What was the matter with me? This cannot be normal.

Intent on isolating myself with each milestone and prognosis that came along, I wanted to share less and less of the experience with my blog readers. I absolutely did not want to post any news on my social media, and I was in no mood to answer my phone to hear yet another excited voice in my ear.

When the radiation treatments ended, I was mentally and physically exhausted. I survived and everyone believed it was the final blow. No way that nightmarish treatment had not killed all the remaining cancer. Except there was one very tiny bee buzzing in my bonnet.

"Do you think I can get Dr. Quilici to take out my other ovary?" I asked Louis one morning while we were on a hike to get my body moving again. Two weeks post radiation, the severe diarrhea had stopped, and I was eating again; it was time to get active and officially begin my recovery.

"Surgeons don't just remove organs because a patient asks them to," Louis responded. And he was right. I had no concrete reason to ask about taking the ovary out. The left ovary was a casualty of my initial surgery in December—it had blown up to the size of a grapefruit from a metastasis of the colon cancer and needed to be removed. Chemotherapy had thrown my right ovary into menopause, and radiation promised to make that permanent. Even so, I never felt good about having the one ovary hanging out in my pelvis.

"Well, I'm going to ask him, anyway. You never know, right?" I called back to him.

The day I stop being stubborn is the day Louis needs to worry that something is seriously wrong. "You never know," he reluctantly echoed. He was walking the trail behind me, but I am certain he was shaking his head and rolling his eyes.

For the next three weeks, having my right ovary removed was all I could talk about. I had a PET scan which showed no signs of hypermetabolic activity (a marker for cancer cells) in my pelvis, liver, or anywhere else in my body. The radiation seemed to have worked, according to the scan. It was time to face Dr. Quilici's pre-op appointment ahead of the reversal and ask him my very important, very cheeky question about removing the ovary.

Dr. Quilici stood across from his assistant, Tiffany, who was at the computer typing his notes, the three of us forming a triangle in the small exam room. The two of them looked intensely at each other. I glanced between them from my perch on the exam table. The silence lasted longer than I had expected, so I was preparing for his negative response and devising my unprofessional rebuttal—I simply planned to burst into tears and make a scene.

"I don't see why not. Add salpingo-oophorectomy to the list," he finally decided. "You're done having children?" he asked, needing official confirmation of that which he already knew.

I made a big production out of puffing air through my lips. "My son is 21, and I just survived Stage-4 colon cancer. I need a baby like I need a hole in the head!" They both chuckled, but my giggles were more from relief than anything else.

The morning after my reversal surgery, both Dr. Quilici and Dr. Jacobs were certain that I was disease free. Dr. Quilici had used the laparoscope to look at my entire abdomen, "Except behind your lungs," and saw no signs of disease, corroborating the recent PET results. Dr. Quilici, in so many ways, had proven himself much more valuable than any PET or CT scan I had had. I left the hospital in disbelief at my good fortune.

"*Technically*, I'm disease free," I would tell my friends and family, updating them on the results of the surgery during the next few days. The extra word was my security blanket, absolving me from having to celebrate anything. I was, of course, relieved that there was no visible disease inside of me, but I was also suspicious. They had not yet posted the pathology report to my hospital portal. Seeing the report myself would allow me to breathe again.

It was natural that everyone around me wanted to cheer the good news. "You're cancer free!" I heard this line so many times, I was convinced it would become a jinx. "He said *disease*-free, not *cancer*-free," I corrected the excited voices on the other end of the phone.

I relished in the knowledge of saying this less to protect myself and more to trample other people's happiness. Being a killjoy was giving me immense amounts of dark pleasure.

In the early days of my recovery, I was diligent about following the "soft solids" diet my nutritionist had prescribed, afraid of taxing my delicate healing insides by introducing new foods too soon. It was difficult to put enough calories in me to regain the pounds I lost during the hospital stay. Since radiation ended, I could not gain a single pound no matter how much or what sorts of foods I ate. I was eighteen pounds lighter than I had been one year ago. My jeans were hanging off me, making my weight loss look exaggerated; not being able to wear my own clothes frustrated me. Buying new jeans in a smaller size a few weeks after surgery made me feel better about my changed body.

"This is just what you weigh now," my primary physician, Dr. Kagan, said to me at my post-op physical. "You're eating well, your reversal is working, and you're feeling good. Don't stress yourself out over your weight." He was right. The more I worried about my weight, the harder it was to eat. Besides, I had lost muscle mass to the cancer. That takes a lot more effort to rebuild than just gaining fat.

Dr. Quilici had also warned me not to do any yoga for eight weeks post-op as the risk of a hernia through the newly closed stoma was very high. Although every instinct was screaming for me to get back on the mat, I was serious about following his instructions.

I was not interested in spending much time focused on the supposed good news. Sometimes it would creep into my head despite my best efforts to ignore it. "You don't have cancer anymore..." a little voice would whisper. But it just seemed so unreal, I could not allow myself to accept it. I had spent the last year with cancer. Expecting to turn my way of thinking completely on its heel was like trying to convince myself the sky was orange.

"*Technically*, I'm disease free," I was also correcting myself. A battle was raging between the two hemispheres of my brain. One side was convinced I was healthy and could get back to the business of living. While the other side remained convinced there had to be some cancer still hiding out inside of me, too small for anyone to see.

When I got the notification that they had posted the pathology results to the portal, I was excited. Finally, I had my proof: I was not cancer free. There would be more treatments. I was right all along. The notes may have been technical in their language, but the news I was waiting for was crystal clear: *Ovary with residual metastatic adenocarcinoma of colorectal origin associated with fibrosis and reactive changes consistent with therapy effect.*

A-ha! I was right: I was *not* cancer free. Although technically *now* I was cancer free since Dr. Quilici had removed that particular bit of cancer during surgery. But still! I had been right not to celebrate. I took odd comfort in this twisted medical version of "I told you so."

And not so deep down, it pleased me to know I might have more treatments.

"What compelled you to ask me to remove the ovary?" Dr. Quilici asked at my post-op appointment. "Because what I saw was a perfectly normal ovary other than showing signs that radiation had been applied to it. I would not have removed it if you hadn't asked."

Would Dr. Quilici believe all the weird things that happened to me during treatments? "Well," I started, measuring his potential open-mindedness. "During all my treatments, I received a lot of strange messages from the Universe. I just learned to listen." I was certain he was working out the technical description of an insanity diagnosis. His eyes never left me, and he made no move to interrupt me, so I continued. "And for whatever reason, that ovary kept popping into my head. I just decided I needed to ask you if you could take it out."

He nodded. "That may have been the best decision of your life. That cancer would have become a very serious problem in about six months from now." He patted me on the shoulder and said his familiar line, "You did good, young lady." I felt like a collie who had not chewed his slippers, but instead alerted him to the boy trapped in the well.

The more difficult discussion was yet to come. Tomorrow, I would see Dr. Jacobs and find out what he had planned for me.

"We're going to put you back on Xeloda along with an infusion of Avastin," Dr. Jacobs explained. "I know you had a difficult time with Xeloda before, but that was more likely because of the combination with radiation. We'll start you on it again and just see how it goes."

I felt like I was being handed a set of shiny new training wheels for my racing bike. Even though I could ride well, they would give me one last line of protection and build my confidence. I was more worried about being told no more treatments than about the cancer in my ovary.

In Dr. Jacobs' words, we were "hedging our bets" for a full recovery by attacking any cancer cells that might still be floating around inside of me, small enough to go undetected by my scans.

During the car ride home, Louis was uncharacteristically quiet. I spent the ride staring out the side window, confusing emotions streaked by like the trees along the side of the bleak freeway. Still lost in my reverie, he finally broke the silence. "How do you feel about this?"

"I feel ok about it," I answered. "But I feel..." I hesitated, wondering how I would explain this so that he could understand the complexity.

"...happy there're more drugs?" he finished my thought.

I nodded. "That's weird, right? I feel like I'm supposed to be upset about this, but I'm not. I'm relieved. I was afraid treatment might be over." The hills in the distance were mesmerizing; they never changed, no matter what we discussed on our multitude of trips on this same freeway. "I wasn't ready to be done."

We drove on in silence. If I was struggling to sort out my thoughts, then certainly Louis was having trouble inside his own head. Later that afternoon, I found him sitting alone on the patio, staring out at the mountains just beyond our neighborhood. "I'm exhausted for you," he said quietly. "I had really hoped that this was over."

This had been a tough year for him, taking care of me through the worst months of our lives. I was exhausted for *him*, not myself. I knew I could keep going, taking whatever medicine Dr. Jacobs prescribed next. But I felt guilty knowing that Louis was required to keep going as well. As we had before, we would just plow forward into this next phase of treatment. Our eyes focused on the narrow path, we would place one shaky foot in front of the other no matter how many nettles and thistles might scratch our ankles.

Two weeks later, my first bottle of Xeloda arrived by courier on our doorstep. Every twelve hours, I would take three of the large, light pink, oblong tablets. The three-week cycle consisted of taking the pills for fourteen days, followed by seven days off the drug. Then, I would start the three-week cycle all over again. I would have to wait until I fully healed from the surgery before beginning the Avastin. There was no need to rush to schedule time at the infusion center.

Ahead of my first dose, working out the logistics of taking pills in the morning and evening provided a welcome distraction.

What time would I take each dose? Would I just take them with breakfast and dinner? What would I eat when I took the pills? A full meal was not a requirement. If I took the pills at bedtime, I would just have to have a substantial snack. None of this really mattered. It was just a distraction, something to focus on that amounted to nothing of importance. I hated the idea that these pills were still chemotherapy. If I could distract myself with useless wonderings, then I could live in ignorance a little longer.

Still, I was happy to take the drugs. We were actively continuing my treatments against The Abdominable, and I felt comforted. Soon, I would perform during the holiday season, getting back into my old life.

I was firmly in The Bright. And ready for anything.

Prodigy

Clearly, playing the piano was all fun and games involving making jokes as you fall off the piano bench in front of laughing audiences. I was barely 4 years old. Victor Borge was on Sesame Street, and I was mesmerized.

I loved to be the center of attention, whether that was singing songs I would make up on the spot into my father's tape recorder or demanding at family holiday parties everyone gather around to watch me make up a dance to "Rockin' Around the Christmas Tree." I was always the star of the show. And if I was not, I would inject myself into that role.

Here was something new: the piano. I became obsessed with the giant concert grand pianos Borge played on my tv screen. Emulating my new piano hero, I pretended to put on a seat belt when I sat down for dinner. My father seemed to understand the growing obsession, and we would watch the Victor Borge PBS specials together. Although I did not know how to read yet, I understood that flipping the music upside down on the piano was a pretty funny joke. I was going to be the next one to do it in front of my very own laughing audience.

I pestered my parents to let me take piano lessons. We did not have a piano, but my friend who lived next door did. Her grandmother, who sometimes let me touch the keys when I was over there for playdates, offered to give me piano lessons for free that summer. I was so young that I was learning to read music at the same time I was learning to read words. Practicing between lessons was impossible since we did not have a piano at our house. Being a creative kid, I drew a piano keyboard with crayons on a piece of cardboard and pretended that was my piano. Even with this tremendous disadvantage, I was racing through all the music books that she gave me. She was patient and amused by this precocious youngster, and quickly realized I was no regular 4-year-old. By the time autumn rolled around, she was telling my parents they needed to buy me a real piano and to find a teacher who could properly nurture my obvious talent.

Whatever the grownups were planning behind the scenes was outside my awareness. But months later, on a snowy winter afternoon, my parents took me to a music store and let me loose in the showroom. Walking around the store and playing on all the pianos was like a dream come true. Of course, I went straight for the shiny black grand pianos like Borge played.

A very pretty woman sat down next to me—I wanted to show her all the things I had already learned in my lessons. Playing songs from memory, I aimed to impress her. I even tried out my childish version of piano humor by pretending to sprain my fingers in the hard sections; I was delighted, of course, when she laughed. She patted my back when we were finished and told me she looked forward to seeing me at my first lesson. One week later, I was over the moon when a real piano was being hoisted up the stairs into our second-floor living room. The movers had barely set down the bench before my little butt was on it. I spent the rest of the day playing through all the music I knew.

My very own piano! I promised my parents I would practice every day. I excelled at the piano, but as the music became more difficult, it was clear my hands would not grow big enough. No matter how hard I worked to stretch my hands, I could never reach the big chords needed to play the more advanced music.

Sticking with the piano no longer made sense. For the last few years of my piano studies, I was splitting my practice time, and my heart, with a shinier instrument.

I was young enough when I picked up the flute that it was hardly a tragedy to step away from the piano. The flute was a fun instrument that amused me for a couple of years. I was instantly the best musician in our 4th grade band, and by the 5th grade, I was playing better than most of the kids at the junior high school. No surprise that I grew bored with it and stopped practicing. By the time I was in 8th grade, I was misbehaving in band rehearsals, not practicing my music, and as a result, slipped from first to third chair. When you are the best at something, you always have a bullseye on your back. Another, more ambitious and devoted player is quietly working their butt off to beat you. That was the life lesson I was being taught, but at 13, I was too ambivalent to care.

One Friday after rehearsal, my band teacher pulled me in to her office. She wanted to know what was going on with my bad attitude. "I want to play solos," I told her. This was the undiluted truth; I had the heart of a diva.

"I see," she said. She grew quiet. After a few moments, she disappeared through the mysterious door in the band room that was always locked. When she reappeared, she was holding a small, square, black case. "Here," she said, with a hint of amusement. "If you can figure out how to play this, you'll have more solos than you can count."

I accepted the new instrument and asked if I could play it in band rehearsal on Monday. I clearly remember the charmed look on her face as she handed me a beat-up music book. "You are more than welcome to play it in band on Monday," she chuckled.

Saturday morning, I read the opening pages of the book—which explained how to hold the tiny double reed in your mouth—and dove right in. I was certain that by the end of the weekend, I would wrangle this new instrument. Then, I would be the only kid in the school who played oboe. I would have all the solos to myself, and no matter how I played, no one would be able to steal my seat.

I showed up to band rehearsal on Monday morning, pleased that I now sat in the center chair in the front row, directly under the conductor. Not even my best friend knew what was going on. Lori eyed me from her seat in the clarinet section and mouthed, "What is that?" I silently mouthed back, "An elbow!" We stifled our laughter behind our music stands.

The band played; I counted out rests leading up to the word *solo* in tiny lettering over a few of the notes. As my debut neared, I lifted the instrument and carefully placed the delicate reed on my lower lip exactly the way the book had instructed. I had not had a lesson from my teacher yet; there was no telling what sort of noise was about to erupt out of the instrument. But that did not dampen my enthusiasm. I was filled with courage and assuredness. My teacher's face showed that she, too, was unsure of what was about to happen. Yet she maintained an admirable air of professionalism. Glancing down at me, she whispered, "Ready?" as if this were the most normal thing in the world. I nodded, and she gave the cue for my first oboe solo ever: *c-b-b-c*—the four notes heard 'round the world.

Violently Sad

During chemotherapy, shaving my head was a gigantic step toward accepting the new path I was on. Hair holds trauma, and I was releasing my identity from my former life, the Before Times, when cancer did not exist. I started my road to recovery with a smooth head, each new inch of hair growth representing time passing on this path. Fawning over my new hair was an important step in releasing the huge trauma of cancer. I could feel the weight of that dark energy leaving me.

Although my doctors and nurses hinted I would need help to face the aftereffects of cancer, I figured I could put off finding a therapist. I believed being conscious of the potential problem meant I was already ahead of the game, so I could postpone getting help. I was cocky and flexing my post-cancer recovery, enjoying the surge of energy. Convinced that I was doing great, I wanted to prove to myself I was not like other people. Because I was strong, and I could do this alone.

Sometimes my reflection in the mirror shakes her head at me and I say to her, "What the fuck happened to us?" Unbelievable: *I had cancer!* My body healed, but my mind could not grasp that the thing had happened at all. As the new year ticked by and significant anniversaries appeared on the calendar—diagnosis, start of chemo, end of chemo, surgery, start of radiation, end of radiation—the details were growing less clear in my mind's eye. This thing had happened to me. There were nearly a dozen scars to prove it, but it felt like an almost forgotten dream. Dissolving hummingbirds in their nests.

Sometimes I felt angry, but not because I had cancer; it had more to do with the lasting effects cancer left on me. This makes anger an emotion that I can cope with, so it dissipates quickly. If I learned anything since my diagnosis, it's that anger is a simple emotion, with simple solutions. The other emotions I experience are more complicated to deal with. Even joy is decorated with little sparkles of sadness. In fact, everything I feel, even the positive emotions, is always lit against a backdrop of sadness. If I was going to be honest about what was happening inside my head, then I had to accept that sadness was the root of everything I felt now.

It was not uncommon for me to cry for no reason. I expected these sorts of outbursts to have ended with each successive negative PET-CT result, or during the months when my CEA remained stable. Would I just brush the cancer dirt off my skinned knees and go on with my life like nothing ever happened? I was going to have to learn to live with the permanent angry red scars and figure out how to bounce back from every ding and scrape cancer threw my way. My abdominal skin was tight, my belly button misshapen, and my pubic hair grew unevenly on either side of the midline incision. When I showed it to her, Suzy called it "Cubist Pubis," giving me permission to laugh at how ridiculous it all was. There had to be a way to be ok with wearing all those scars and changes. I needed to be brave enough to look at them while not plotting ways to fix them. It helped me to lift my shirt and show my girlfriends all the surgical scars. Amazingly, they would lift their shirts to show me their various scars, most of which had faded, and tell me how they barely remember what it had been like in the days after those painful surgeries.

But what about the emotional side? I had always used yoga as an emotional outlet beginning 25 years ago when I bought my first yoga book and tried to imitate the photos in my apartment's spare bedroom. I tried yoga as a stress reliever when I was 24 years old and working a job I really had no passion for—teaching general music to middle school students. It was a thankless and stressful job. Besides the overwhelming daily paperwork, it was also physically hazardous—an 8th grade girl hit me in the face when I asked for her hall pass. I spent the year counting the days until June, when I could quit. It was during this year of discontent that yoga appeared to me, offering me some stress-relief, and I accepted the challenge. Yoga was there during my pregnancy. It was there to help me cope with my divorce, and it was there to build my body before and after my cancer diagnosis. I had experienced its benefits multiple times during my life, so it was only natural that I would lean on it now as I tried to emerge from my cancer-cocoon.

Yoga was very different and very difficult after radiation. I would have to accept the changes in my body. My ego struggled to face the fact that in the months just prior to my diagnosis, my body had been at its strongest, most fit, most flexible, most advanced point ever. I could finally do poses that I had spent years working on. And now, post-cancer, I had lost so much ground. The skin of my abdomen was so tight from all the surgeries that sometimes I felt as if I were wearing an unyielding leather bodysuit. It was nearly impossible to reach my toes now, and my shoulders resisted just about every movement. Some poses required modifications, forcing me to experiment with variations, all to accommodate my new body. At first, I was resentful that cancer forced me into these changes. The easy path was paved in anger, but compassion would be the only way to accept my new post-cancer body.

No amount of self-realization could prepare me for the waves of emotion that crashed over me sometimes. Ustrasana, commonly called Camel Pose, is known among yogis as a heart opener. To do the pose, you stand on your knees, bend backwards, reach down for your heels, arch your back, and lift your heart to the sky. With your head tipped back in a most vulnerable position, you offer your soft throat to the world. Yoga teachers always explain in classes how this advanced pose opens energy channels in the front of the body, which are often blocked because we protect our chests and bellies like dogs. In back-bending poses, we need to breathe and allow the energy to flow. There is no way of knowing what sort of energy we will release. We just have to let it happen. If we can observe our reaction to the experience, then we learn important lessons about ourselves. Camel pose, to a higher degree than many other backbends, forces me to be an active participant in my emotional healing. This was made more difficult with the shadow of cancer looming over me.

My knees firmly planted on the mat, my hands pressed gently into my lower back to nudge my hips forward. I lifted my chest and arched back, finding a spot to look at on the ceiling as I released my hands and reached down for my heels. My straightened arms balanced my backward leaning, their strength helped me push past what had been a stiff arch to ease my body into a half moon shape. At first, I was relaxed, and breathed as deeply as I could. This pose takes a lot of strength and patience, and every part of my body was quickly tiring with the effort.

And then, it became impossible to take a breath. I let go of my heels and my body flung forward like a bent sapling springing back to vertical. Air suddenly sucking into my lungs, I felt the oncoming explosion hurtling at me like a freight train. The tears were inevitable, but it was the emotion behind them that was staggering. My chest hurt, my face scrunched as if I were feeling agonizing pain, and I let out a sound like a wild animal. In just a few sobs, I realized this cry was going to need help. I pulled myself off the mat, tears streaming down my face, and walked out to the patio where Louis was sipping his coffee.

"Oh no, what's wrong?" He asked. I threw myself down on the sofa next to him and dropped my head onto his chest. Safe in his arms, there was no stopping the waves. "Did something happen?" He stroked my cheek.

"No," I gasped. "I'm just violently sad."

He let me cry until I calmed down, my breathing slowing and body relaxing. "Sadness is the most pervasive emotion in the universe," he explained in his quiet way. "There are horrible things happening in the world right now, and maybe you tapped into that river of sadness, the heartbreak of the planet weeping."

He could be right. The injustice of what we humans do to each other and to the animals and the planet itself affects me deeply. I have cried for slaughtered dolphins, clubbed seals, and abused dogs; starving African children, kidnapped children, and murdered children; battered women, prisoners of war, and people who throw themselves from bridges; and ocean pollution, nuclear meltdowns, and chemical warfare. The world is filled with so much pain and suffering. Sometimes it is too much for me to bear. Cancer has taken what was already a painful awareness and exaggerated it to the point of heartache. I am so acutely aware of these horrible things—how we choose to destroy and consume. We hardly appreciate just how miraculous the planet is—a tiny oasis of life floating helpless and inconspicuous through the vastness of space. I hug trees and lie on the grass. I love the Earth. This would be such a wondrous place to live if more people loved the planet.

"There are so many beautiful things, though," he continued. "Once you feel the sadness, remind yourself of the amazing things you get to experience."

My attention was focused on the leaves on the trees. I imagined all the tiny hummingbird nests hidden in the branches. At least in our backyard, our little, tiny insignificant square of land, no harm comes to any of the creatures who choose to live here. In the universe's vastness, we make no difference. But to the animals that call it home, it means everything. They can live safely and with no cares here, and that is my contribution. If I leave nothing else behind, I hope I have made life just a little easier for the gentle beings in my yard. And with tears still stinging my eyes, I allowed myself to believe my life has served some small purpose.

Part 2

"What does it matter? And why should I care?"
–me

Hz

"Shhhh, shhh, shh....." Louis' voice broke through the sound of scrambling dog nails on the hardwood floor. "You're safe. I'm here. You're in your bed." I grasped on to his shirt, my face buried in his neck, tears streaming from my eyes. My heart was racing. I could barely breathe. I felt as if I would vomit. "Shhh..." he continued to soothe. "You're safe." He chanted the mantra again and again.

My heart was pounding out of my chest, my body shaking uncontrollably. What in the world had just happened? Despite the panic in my body, my mind was grasping desperately at the dream I had just been having. It was, as far as dreams go, the usual jumble of incongruity of pleasant dreams. Nothing scary.

It took a solid five minutes to come down from this fright. Against me, I could feel Louis shaking a little. I had probably scared the shit out of him, waking him from a dead sleep with my shrieking and thrashing.

"That was a good one," he whispered, pressing his hand into my cheek, and kissing the top of my head. "Do you want to talk about it?"

I shook my head. "I don't even remember what happened," I said. We coordinated our breathing so I could slow myself down. Was it a nightmare? Was it a panic attack? Was it something else entirely? My head was foggy. In the background, under the rush of blood pulsing in my eardrums, I could hear the sound bath playing through the speakers. 528Hz was the frequency I had been listening to since I awoke to my diagnosis last year. We listened to it every single night; it had become part of the landscape of our sleeping pattern; sometimes we hardly noticed it anymore. But other times, like right now, I was thankful for the tones and white noise. It was something to anchor to.

"Was it a nightmare?" Louis prompted again. I pressed my head against him, relaxing a bit. He went through a series of questions, hoping to jog my memory and sort out what had happened. Like a forensic dreamologist, he was working his magic in the dark.

Like swirling smoke, things were coming back into focus. I had been dreaming about our dogs and a large parcel of land, probably because of a movie we had watched that evening. In the dream, I had been watching the dogs running through the tall grasses. Through the dream, I heard the 528Hz cutting into my subconscious. It was pleasant and reassuring. It was acting as a trigger to begin lucid dreaming, a skill I had been practicing for decades. The sound of the frequency allowed me to fully experience the dream as a dream, and if I were really in control, I could interact with my dream in some amazing ways.

As I was relaxing into the first stage of my lucidity, something happened. A voice cut through the music, so close to my ear there might have been someone standing next to the bed. Whatever they said was incomprehensible to me; it sounded more like a scream run through a distortion effect. The fright had been so severe that I was in terror, waking Louis, chasing off the dogs, and turning me into a blathering mess. I relayed these things to Louis as we laid there in the dark.

"Maybe you were receiving another message," he suggested. "You were open, and something tried to make contact?"

I shook my head. I sighed. "Maybe. I wish I could have understood what the voice was saying." Perhaps my days of being an open channel to strange realms were ending. Receiving and processing visions and messages might be a thing of the past. This made me a little sad. The last message I received had practically saved my life. I would miss this special connection I had to the unknown and unknowable. From now on, when messages came in, would I react with fright instead of wonderment?

While I was going through chemotherapy, I came to expect strange happenings in the middle of the night. Chemo brought about complicated sleeping patterns. The steroids, which are given to help ease some of the side effects, gave me insomnia. But, in between rounds, they would wear off just enough for me to fall into a deep sleep. During that period I experienced deep delicious sleep, and even when I awakened, I could simply roll over and go back to sleep.

During one of the last rounds of chemo, I had a unique experience—I still do not know if it was real or a hallucination. It began like every other night in what had been a long line of 3:20 a.m. wake-ups.

An irritating pain in my chest from the portacath woke me— my sleeping position was crushing it. The caustic chemotherapy drugs irritated the implant, which left it perpetually sore and uncomfortable. If anything touched it, I would get a slightly nauseous feeling. I could not wait to get this thing taken out of me. I just had to tolerate it through the treatments. Everyone said it would be less irritating after chemo was over. Laying on my right side took all the pressure off the portacath. If I were a little more comfortable, I could sleep. So, I rolled over.

If the dogs heard me moving around, it was only a matter of time before one of them would be up on the bed, sniffing my ear and trying to lick my face. At my slightest noise, Dusty would think that it was time to start the day. After rolling, I tried to lie as still as possible. But it was too late. Someone had jumped up on to the bed and was carefully stepping over my bent legs. I freed my left arm from the blanket and reached out into the darkness. A wet nose pressed against my fingers and acknowledged them with a soft lick. This confirmed my suspicion that it was Dusty; Luna only licks my hand if there is something delicious on it.

I expected the dog would jump back down, having satisfied his curiosity about me being awake. But he did not. Instead, he laid down against my belly, pressing himself as close to me as he could. Dusty is not typically this cuddly; I took advantage of this rare moment of affection. I put my arm over him, my hand snaking in between his front legs and pulling him into a tighter snuggle. He pushed his cold nose into the space between my neck and my pillow, gently nuzzling me. I thought it was pretty cheeky of him to get this comfortable. But ultimately, I was thrilled that my insecure dog wanted to sleep in my arms.

We laid together like that for several minutes, his nose under my neck, my hand stroking his side. I ran my hand down his body, reaching for his tail. Both Dusty and his sister have rigid, curled tails. One hint of their breeding, this tail shape comes from their Basenji father. But this dog's tail was floppy, long, and covered in a fine puff of soft fur.

Who is this? I stayed quiet, continuing to stroke the dog's side, edging my hand up toward their head. I scratched the neck and felt the feet squirm a little. On the head, I felt an ear—a large, strong, pointy ear about the size of my hand. Seriously: *who is this?*

A soft voice near my feet whispered, "Coyote is always with you."

Not frightened at all, I pressed my cheek closer to the wet nose, and the animal licked me softly. I basked in the warmth of the little body next to me. We lay like that for some time. Gradually, the coyote dissolved, leaving my arm hovering just above the blankets, which still radiated the residual warmth of its body. Whether it was a dream or a vision was of little concern. It had happened, and I held onto the message, not knowing its ultimate meaning.

I had had so many of these other-worldly messages from the invisible allies standing watch around my bed, I should have been used to hearing voices in the dark. On this night, the fifth messenger had been trying to speak. But, I had been too scared to listen.

Louis laid awake next to me. Finally calm, I tried to get back to sleep. The 528Hz continued playing, so I latched on to the lowest of the octaves, hearing the pulsing vibrations and feeling them within my cells. It embarrassed me I had rejected the message so violently and hoped that in the future, I would be calm and wise enough to recognize the next one.

Monkey Dish

I expected to take the Xeloda pills and just move on with my life. I began making plans for how I would return to performing, even committing to a holiday concert I was certain I would be ready for. Despite all the medications and severe side effects, I was practicing diligently so that I would be absolutely ready, physically and emotionally, for this concert in December.

I went on an appreciation campaign for everyone who helped me through this tough year. I popped into an orchestra rehearsal to stand on the podium and thank all 75 musicians through a torrent of tears. Ella took me out to lunch a couple of times and Pam indulged me with a day of playing cello in her living room. It was nice to see my friends without the specter of cancer hanging over me. Even though I was *technically* disease free, everyone was treating me as if I was *literally* cancer free, and it felt great. If my trusted support crew continued to push this perspective, then the higher the probability I might eventually believe it.

After my reversal surgery, I spent quite some time trying to figure out how to close out my blog. I needed to relieve myself of further responsibility to continue to post these updates. I felt a great deal of pressure to maintain the weekly posts. Although adjuvant chemotherapy treatments were going to continue for at least another year, there was no need for me to write about it. None of the doctors expected me to experience the same level of physical or mental strain that I had already experienced with FOLFIRINOX. It was time for me to slip back into a private life and enjoy anonymity again. Besides, maintenance chemo was not as glamorous as real chemo; who would be interested in this part, anyway?

"This is called a monkey dish," I informed Louis. "And I stole it from the restaurant where I worked in back in 1996," I confessed with all the pride of an evil mastermind.

The three pink Xeloda pills laid at the bottom of the stolen dish, which I happily held out for his inspection. Because chemotherapy can be toxic through the skin, the pharmacist told me not to hold the pills in my hands or mouth for too long. This was why I was serving up the pills in a fancy antique dish this morning.

I wished the pills good luck, placed the first one carefully on the back of my tongue, and quickly swallowed it with a mouthful of water. For no particular reason, it became increasingly difficult to swallow each subsequent pill. I chalked it up to a mental block.

While I was on radiation three months earlier, Dr. Jacobs had prescribed this same drug. As the weeks pressed on, it became difficult to disentangle the effects of the drug from those of the radiation treatments. They seemed to influence each other, weaving a tangled web of issues that were amplifying those of the other in dangerous ways. The diarrhea could have been a side effect of either the Xeloda or the IMRT. No matter from which it originated, by the end of treatments, it left me dangerously dehydrated, causing my blood pressure to drop. Nausea was a side effect of both the drug and the radiation. Xeloda was there to enhance the effect of the radiation on all my cells, whether cancerous or healthy, and it was taking its job seriously. I gave up trying to sort it all out, and eventually Dr. Jacobs took me off the drug so that I might survive the final ten doses of radiation.

But this time around, there would be no other treatment along with the Xeloda to exaggerate its side effects. No more radiation to blame. I would feel the full unfiltered effects of the Xeloda and know for certain it was the culprit.

Dr. Jacobs began by prescribing six pills, 3000 mg, per day. The first dose made me disinterested in anything that required standing up from the sofa. My energy had dialed down, giving me a bad case of couch lock. I had nausea and acid reflux again, so it was time to dig out the leftover Zofran and Prilosec from the bottom of my medicine drawer. I was caught up, yet again, in Xeloda's clutches. It was clear the drug and my digestive tract would never play nice together.

My hands and feet reacted to the drug. Hand and Foot Syndrome, my old friend, was back in full force. My hands were bright red, swollen, and stiff. Chemo often takes a year to clear out of the body. It was why I still had neuropathy from the Oxaliplatin and dry skin from the 5-Fluorouracil (5-FU) seven months after primary chemotherapy had ended. Xeloda is 5-FU in pill form, so since I was adding more of this drug into my already flooded system, we expected that the familiar side effects would reappear quickly.

My feet were worse and harder to deal with than my hands. Unless I felt like hobbling around on my knees or forcing Louis to carry me everywhere, using my feet was unavoidable. Huge chunks of skin were breaking off and peeling from my toes; the soles felt as if they were burnt on hot coals and covered by wool socks. Walking, hiking, running, yoga—anything that required the use of my feet—was off the table. I needed to rest and wait for my next check-up with Dr. Jacobs.

"This is why I wanted to see you after one round of the drug," he told me, turning my hands over in his to examine my red, swollen fingers and inflamed palms. I knew him well enough now to recognize the shape his eyebrows were making over his mask. He was worried. He dropped my daily dosage to four pills, 2000 mg, hoping my hands and feet would get better.

My training wheels had been installed on a bike that threatened to fall apart at every turn. Still, the side effects were more than expected, so again, he dropped the dosage. Now, I was down to just two pills, 1000 mg, per day—such a low dose that we all wondered if it would actually have any effect on residual cancer cells. This low dose would surely help my hands, or at least get them to a point I could live with. I bargained for more time on the higher dosage. Dr. Jacobs was unmoved. "We don't want you to end up with an infection in your hands," he said, tracing a deeply cracked line in my palm which had opened up to reveal the tender pink lower layers of skin.

My hands were not nearly as bad as they were during chemotherapy last spring, but they were preventing me from playing my cello, practicing yoga, and doing basic things around the house. They were swollen, burned, and cracked, and I was frustrated.

No way would my hands heal in time. I would have to back out of the December concert. Even though my hands were literally shredding to pieces, strips of skin hanging from between my fingers, and the palms filled with cracks and open wounds, I still hesitated to make the call to tell the other musicians I could not play. Admitting it would be physically impossible felt like a bigger deal than it was in actuality. My colleagues had been *hopeful* I would join them, nothing more. They were always cautious with how much they encouraged me. It seemed like everyone was operating in a more sober version of my reality than I was.

I would have to be on adjuvant therapies for at least a year, maybe even as long as three years. But the first six weeks had made us all question if I could take the drug for that long. Dr. Jacobs suggested we might change back to 5-FU, controlling the exact dosage with the infused version may spare my hands. The pill form had promised convenience. Instead, I might have 5-FU infusions every third week as well. Getting to see the infusion nurses was a silver lining, though.

But first, Dr. Jacobs decided I needed a break from the Xeloda. Hopefully, during this extra week without the drugs, my hands would heal. At the very least, my energy level would come back up so I would be strong and ready to face the upcoming infusions. Louis and I decided that during this break, we needed a vacation. For months, he had gone out to lunch with his sons and met with colleagues and clients. He had been all over the greater Los Angeles area while I had quarantined in the house. The only places I went to were the hospital, cancer center, and doctors' appointments. I was tired of these walls. What was the purpose in surviving if I was going to be under indefinite house arrest?

We took a trip to Monterey, California. This is a special place for us. We have vacationed there too many times to count; the first time while we were dating. He had been right in assuming I would love the cloudy skies and stormy seas of California's mid-coast. We spent our honeymoon there, drinking wine on the balcony, watching the otters in the bay, and waking to the barking of harbor seals on the rocks below our room each sunrise. I was looking forward to this trip. I packed my bag a week ahead of our departure, carefully planned my wardrobe, and made a mental map to navigate through the aquarium. The vacation proved useful. I felt invigorated. Staring out at the ocean for many uninterrupted hours each day prepared me to take on this next treatment phase.

Avastin was the second drug to be added to my adjuvant treatment. It is supposed to be a part of the FOLFIRINOX regimen, but because I was still recovering from the colectomy, they did not include it in my original treatment. I needed to wait three months after my reversal surgery to start the drug infusions. That was fine with me. Even though I saw the maintenance drugs as an emotional crutch, it still felt good to postpone. I was happy for any break in this long line of treatments. Now that I had the freedom of life on Xeloda, I wanted to enjoy it; I was not champing at the bit to get back to the infusion center for anything.

My CEA (carcinoembryonic antigen) was of particular interest to me, as this is used to monitor my progress during treatments. Not used to diagnose any specific cancer, CEA levels can rise if cancer, or certain non-cancerous conditions, are present. In a normal, non-smoking adult, the level of CEA should be less than 5.0 nanograms per milliliter (ng/mL). In my case, at the time of my diagnosis in 2021, my CEA measured 13.1 ng/mL. Obviously, it was elevated because I had cancer. Immediately following my colectomy, during which a large amount of the primary cancer was removed, my CEA had a sharp decrease. During chemotherapy treatments, Dr. Jacobs checked my CEA periodically over those twelve weeks. As expected, my CEA fluctuated a bit during that time, which, as he explained to me, was a result of my body's natural response to the drugs. It did not mean cancer was growing or worsening. Still, I worried.

Weekly blood test results were becoming my obsession. Although I had very little understanding of what I was looking at in the CBC (Complete Blood Count) or the Basic Metabolic Panel, I kept note of trends in my white and red blood cell counts, eGFR (kidney function), and of course the CEA.

With low white blood cells, I was always at a greater risk of infection. I was diligent in wearing a surgical mask everywhere I went. Everyone else was loosening up and not wearing masks as the COVID pandemic lost steam—people were losing patience and interest in following whatever guidelines lingered. But the virus was still out there, showing up as new variants. It was not unusual for me to be the only person wearing a mask in a restaurant or store. I got plenty of sideways looks from strangers. Mask wearing had become oddly political during the pandemic, a divisive identifier instead of being viewed as protection from the disease. Again, I toyed with shaving my head: if I were bald, people may not question why I was wearing a mask. Now that I was sporting a traditional short haircut, I was subjected to the dirty looks yet again. But I did not care. This was a matter of life and death, not politics. Even a common cold could turn critical for me. The timing of my cancer diagnosis and treatments meant I did not get any of the COVID vaccine boosters, only the initial doses in 2021. None of that was anyone's business at the grocery store.

Just before beginning radiation, I was thrilled to see my lowest CEA result ever: 1.8 ng/mL. This was the first time my numbers were well beneath the minimum. I was feeling pleased and quite full of myself. But with radiation, the CEA fluctuated yet again. During breaks from treatment, my CEA would fall; it would rise when they resumed. I was driving myself crazy following these numbers. At the same time, I was learning a lot about how my body reacted to each new thing that was thrown at it.

Having learned all about my CEA during the previous ten months of treatments, I should not have been as surprised as I was to see my CEA climb after my colostomy reversal surgery in September. As expected, it rose slightly in the weeks immediately after. Eight weeks later, when I began taking the new Xeloda prescription, my CEA suddenly shot up to 7.5 ng/mL.

There was no reason, other than curiosity, for me to be poking around in my medical portal for the CEA results. I could have—and probably should have—just waited for Dr. Jacobs to inform me on a need-to-know basis. But since I had little else to distract me these days, scaring myself gave me something to do. My old friend insomnia reared its ugly head at night, and during the day I was anxious and moody. Between visits with Dr. Jacobs, the one person who could explain the results in a way that gave me hope instead of terror, I had plenty of time to imagine the worst.

Louis tried, and sometimes succeeded, to convince me that there was no way cancer would regrow so quickly. It was impossible that Dr. Quilici had seen no visible signs of disease in September, and then new cancer would grow out of control in a matter of weeks, raising the CEA in November. It had to be a fluke. Louis was certain Dr. Jacobs would tell me as much. Sitting in the exam room listening to Dr. Jacobs do exactly what Louis had predicted, my eyes still stung with tears.

"We don't use the CEA for diagnosis. With you, we're just looking at the trends." He was well aware of my teary eyes and gave my hand a warm squeeze. "You'll see: the numbers will trend downward soon enough." He reassured me that this was all expected, but he would order the test more often so I could see those numbers heading back in the right direction.

Has Dr. Jacobs ever been wrong? He has always seen the bigger picture while I was focused on the minutia, and it was important for me to remember that. He should wear one of those *Bomb Squad: if you see me running, try to keep up* T-shirts because I should know by now that unless I see him panicking, then there is nothing to worry about.

I had no frame of reference, though, what a frightening CEA was. I was working within such a small range that I lost sight of how high this number can climb. Talking with other colorectal cancer patients, I discovered that some were getting readings closer to 2000 ng/mL, which put my worries about 7.5 ng/mL into perspective. I was working myself up over (literally) nothing; no wonder Dr. Jacobs was looking at me with warm amusement.

"I know we're splitting hairs," I said to him.

He laughed. "Yes, but it's a very fat hair and we don't want to see it hit five."

As the weeks went on, the numbers crept back down to a comfortable place. A little slower than I might have liked, but they were definitely going in the right direction. In my case, having unfettered access to my blood test results and medical notes has proven to cause more stress than necessary. Dr. Jacobs must tire of inquisitive patients without a medical degree, like me, obsessing over test results they did not understand.

On the one-year anniversary of my very first FOLFIRINOX chemotherapy, the 3-month waiting period to begin the Avastin expired, and I was back in the infusion center for my first treatment. I tried not to put too much importance on this scheduling coincidence. I did not know what this drug would do to me. Dr. Jacobs and the nurses were constantly reassuring me, "This is nothing." Still, I could not prevent the little tendrils of fear from twisting in my brain. Any drug with the label chemotherapy attached to it would elicit a powerful reaction from anyone.

At the infusion center that morning, I felt like it was the first day of 10th grade: with one year of experience under my belt, I knew what to expect and where to go. I was looking forward to seeing everyone again, yet nervous about the new drug. Abby spent a lot of time sitting with me in my cubicle, catching up with me. The last time she had seen me was for hydration treatments six months ago during radiation. She had never met me when I was healthy. It was fun to get to know each other again, this time as I really am.

"Do you remember why we put chemo drugs in the brown cover?" Abby asked as she hung the little bag of Avastin from my IV tree.

"Yes! That's the UV light cover," I answered. I am the star student no matter where I go.

She laughed. "Very good! When can you start work? We're shorthanded."

"Believe me, I'm so squeamish, I'd probably pass out the first time I had to poke someone's portacath." After laughing and exchanging stories of some of the more gross things we have witnessed with pets and kids, she accessed my portacath and began administering the drug. This infusion would only take twenty minutes. That was hardly enough time to crack open a book. Louis and I texted with each other, even though we were sitting just three feet apart.

"Can you feel anything from the drug?" Louis asked. He looked at me as if he expected something dramatic to happen. So, I indulged him by making some humorous choking noises while wagging my head from side to side. Concluding with a dramatic slump, I let my tongue loll out. I waited a few seconds before I cracked one eye to peek at him; I needed to be sure he had seen my performance.

"I should have known better." He rolled his eyes at me and went back to his crossword.

Dark Wavy Cloud

I was 48 years old, but I looked and felt like I was 60. No one agreed with me: most people told me I looked better than they remembered. My stepson, Benjamin, had said I looked "Alive again." I so badly wanted to believe him. The last time many of my friends and colleagues had seen me was in the weeks before my diagnosis. During that time, even while dressed up for concerts and wearing makeup, it was hard to hide the fact that I looked drawn, tired, worried, and thin. A picture from a concert one month before my diagnosis makes it difficult to deny that my hair looks dull and scraggly; my face looks wrinkled and leathery; my eyes look distant and unfocused; even my teeth look disinterested in participating in the photo. Compared to that, of course I looked great now.

A photo that Louis took while we were hiking during chemo gave me some insight into what I should expect to look like when I really am 60. Overall, not bad. But at 48, I am still in the pocket where the last traces of youth might outshine some new grey hairs and the tiny crow's feet. I appreciated why actresses feel they need plastic surgery. Post-treatments, I was secretly contemplating getting Botox in my brow and I am hardly a pop culture icon who has to live up to a signature look.

My friend Ella, who went through chemotherapy and radiation for her cancer nearly fourteen years ago, reminded me that the treatments change our bodies in ways that can never be fixed. I understood the cause behind the changes. What I refused to accept was that some wounds may never heal. If I had my way, I would be back to my old self, no matter how many times everyone told me it was impossible.

There was plenty of scar tissue leftover in my pelvis after radiation treatments, which left me with a slight limp. After many weeks and months of yoga practice, I saw some real physical improvements. If that was how much I could fix my hips in six months, then I had every reason to believe that, with a year of hard work and recovery, the improvements would be even more extensive and obvious. Being able to put my feet behind my head again might seem like a useless skill in the grand scheme of things, but it represented an increased range of motion. If I could do that, then theoretically, there were no limits to how much I could heal my body.

When I looked in the mirror, I thought I looked just fine. I am not delusional and expect to look like I did in my 30s. But overall, I had no complaints about my new reflection. My skin looked softer because there was some fat under the surface again. Without ovaries and hormones, I had no rogue pimples. Although I weighed 16-pounds less than I normally did, it seemed to make no difference to my overall healthy appearance. It was my perception that was important. As long as I stuck to mirror gazing, where I could pose in more flattering angles, I felt just fine about my new, more mature, look.

In a startling blow to my ego, Louis took some pictures of me on Christmas morning. We wanted to celebrate the insane victory of living a year past my diagnosis. I sat in front of the Christmas tree, wearing the plaid one-piece pajamas he had given me, and flashed a big goofy grin with a thumbs up. Through all my treatments, the joke was that I sent Lori "Fonzie" photos from scary places—getting a chemotherapy infusion, laying inside the radiation machine, on the gurney headed for a surgery. It allowed me to laugh through the dark moments. I would flash a thumbs up while sitting behind all my medications lined up on the table or laying in my hospital bed post-op, and suddenly I was less terrified, too. On Christmas morning, we took another thumbs up photo, this time without the irony: it was time to celebrate the year.

"What the hell?" I demanded of Louis when he showed me the results of our photo shoot.

He laughed and told me to stop being so hard on myself. "It's just a couple of grey hairs," he reassured me. "And the lighting is weird."

No. It was not the grey hairs or the lighting that made the picture weird. "What happened to my face?" He grew serious when he saw I was on the verge of tears. This unexpected visceral reaction surprised me, too. I blinked back the tears and told him to delete the pictures; we would try again later. Certainly, I would look miraculously younger if I could age another 90 minutes.

"I will do no such thing," he dug in. "I don't know what you're seeing in these photos, but you look healthy and happy. I'm going to keep them for myself even if you don't want them." He turned off his phone and put it in his pocket. Discussion over. "It's not up to you to decide what pictures of my wife I like to look at."

"Ugh," I moaned. "Fine." We were even—I had plenty of pictures of him I loved and which he hated. There was no way I would send any of these pictures to Lori—I was under no marital obligation to her.

"I think you have less grey hair than I remember," Pam said to me a few days later when I visited her house to exchange our gifts. After making this declaration, she reached out and started rifling through my hair—inspecting me like a mamma bear. I laughed as she shooed my hand away. "I'm not seeing as many," she declared, hands on her hips. The look on her face dared me to challenge her.

"Well, ok then." I was relieved of duty. Another woman had given me permission to ignore the parts of my hair not visible in the mirror.

Growing my hair back had turned into a bigger ordeal than I expected. In the early stages, I had a soft carpet of spiky hair that was the same color as Luna's. But she was neither amused nor interested in sitting still for pictures together. My new hair was unique, and sometimes I thought it was pretty.

The months dragged on, and as it grew longer, the strands curled. The joke around the house was that my hair was going through what we called "The Phases of Ross," using his hair styles in *Friends* as colorful descriptions of my current hair style. "I'm Ross-Season 5," I would complain to Lori over texts. Meanwhile, I was trying to tame my unruly mane with various hair products. My hair was so thick it formed itself into a dark, wavy cloud over my head. I hated it. I was looking forward to when my hair might lie down flat, like Monica's super cute haircut in Season 4. I spent too much time imagining my future hair.

"You look so cute with short hair!" Everyone was quick to compliment my new short style. I tried not to be too cynical since they were being genuinely kind. "You should definitely keep it like this for a while," they would advise.

Wistfully staring at old pictures of myself, I missed wearing ponytails and braids, and longed for the feeling of long hair brushing against my neck. None of this was my choice. My hair was short because I had had cancer. It was short because chemo had made it fall out. It was short because something awful had happened to me. And it was sending out mixed messages: on one hand, the recent growth reminded me I was healing, but on the other it reminded me I almost died as an unrecognizable, skinny cancer patient with a bald head.

I was just being impatient. Hiking and yoga were improving my aerobic fitness despite the low red blood cells, and I was coping with the changes in my bowel habits after the reversal. But there was nothing I could do about my hair.

Within nine months, my hair was well on its way to growing out. No longer bald like a cancer patient, or fuzzy like a recovering survivor, I lacked the outward signs of a recent illness. Hard to believe, but I missed the stares I was getting when we went somewhere. There was no emotional middle ground—I either wanted to be bald or have my old hair back. But no matter how petulant I was, I could not force my hair to grow on my schedule.

By the end of the first year, my part had moved back to the correct side of my head and the chemo curls relaxed. By not wearing hats when I was out hiking, my natural color came back quickly. With my fair skin, hazel eyes, and freckles, the lighter hair made me look more familiar to myself again.

I could not help feeling self-conscious, though. Trying everything to put a little style into my hair, I had piles of hair products, gels, pastes, spray wax, and sculpting creams. But, I was no hair stylist—I mostly succeeded in turning my hair into a sticky mess, which molded itself into cartoonish shapes while I slept. It was easier just to hide it with clips and fabric than to style it.

It appeared the cancer and the chemotherapy drugs had loosened their grip on my body. If things like my hair and nails were growing back so fervidly, then it was true: my body was no longer competing with cancer for calories and could waste its energy growing useless decorations again.

While others were celebrating my appearance, I was stressing. But maybe, just maybe, I could see myself through their eyes. Maybe I could appreciate how amazing this transformation was. I am not going back to who I was. I am blossoming into the new person who I am. My new hair can reflect not just my good health, but also my new persona. Short hair may just be a phase that New Lisa has to get through on her journey, but it is certainly teaching me a lot about patience and acceptance.

"Looking like a cancer patient" had been my identity for nearly a year, but that was over. It was time to embrace my new hair and the new attitude having survived cancer gifted me. The distance between myself and cancer was increasing every month that I lived—measured by the length of my hair.

"Can you believe that one year ago, I was bald and had only just finished my third infusion?" I said to Louis as we hiked one chilly Saturday morning in February. Although my red blood cell count was still low, I had somehow adapted to the strain on my lungs and hiked the tough trails with very little discomfort. Not out of breath, I did not need long breaks like I did during chemo. One year ago felt both like a lifetime and the blink of an eye.

Louis had been walking in front of me, leading us through the overgrown trail that was blooming in wildflowers. The cooler temperatures and unusually rainy winter had made the mountain explode in plant life. I had never seen the trails so lush. It was only a matter of time before the Painted Ladies began erupting from their cocoons.

As soon as I spoke, Louis stopped and turned to face me. I was standing above him at the curve of a switchback. "It's really hard to believe," he said, a dark cloud came over his face. "You should be dead right now." My nose was running, not because I was sick, but because the Xeloda affected my sinuses. There was a streak of red on the tissue, and although I tried to hide it, Louis still saw it. His brow furrowed briefly. "And yet, here you are on this mountain on this beautiful day, hiking like nothing even happened."

I knew he was right. That I was acting almost like my old self was a miracle. Something outside the realm of normal had happened here. I made it happen. The doctors made it happen. Louis made it happen. There was nothing supernatural about my survival—they pumped drugs into me, I used all my mental and physical strength to endure the side effects, and ultimately, I won the tug-of-war with Death and got to keep my life for a little longer.

We stood there for several minutes, looking out on the hills below us, trying to identify the other trails carved into the park. An airplane crashed into these mountains in 1949. A cross now stands on the hill marking the place where it happened. It was difficult to see it from where we were standing. We spent a few minutes trying to pick it out among the scrubby trees and rocks below before we found it.

I thought about the people on that ill-fated airplane, wondering if they could see the quickly approaching hills out their windows, their stomachs dropping as the plane lost altitude, knowing death was moments away. Being told I have cancer is about as close to being in a plane crash as I have ever been: the bottom dropped out from under me and the scenery rushed at me faster than I could process. I was powerless as the trees and rocks grew larger through my window, blocking out the sky.

I pulled out of the dive because Dr. Quilici jumped over me to grab the yoke while Dr. Jacobs pulled hard from the right seat; I cowered in the back seat, protecting my head between my knees. They shouted at me and no matter how crazy or scary those instructions were, I followed them; my little plane miraculously skimmed the tops of the trees and gained altitude, finally leveling off and gliding through the blue sky again. All the while, the two pilots up front remained cool.

The Krukenberg Effect

Cancer never quits. Physically and emotionally. Although my body is *technically* disease free, my mind is still being devoured by carcinomas, sarcomas, myelomas, blastomas, and neoplasms. Without the physical symptoms of the colon cancer as a constant reminder of what was going on inside of me, I expected to spend less time thinking about cancer and more time living like a normal person. I was so wrong.

The memory of the surprise cancer hiding out deep inside the right ovary was eating away at my daily joy. The ovary was removed; that cancer was incinerated. I should have nothing to worry about. After dodging the bullet, instead of running off to celebrate, I had tipped over like one of those fainting goats.

There had been cancer hiding inside of me that no one saw. How could I trust any scans ever again? What else was hiding?

"What compelled you to ask me to remove that ovary?" Dr. Quilici asked me at my follow-up appointment after my reversal surgery and the fateful pathology report.

I wish I could claim that I knew it was there, and that was why I had asked him to take it out of me. But that could not be further from the truth. I knew nothing; I was just reacting to a gut feeling with no specific cause. I was simply uneasy and obsessed with The Ovary.

He was not the only doctor interested in my self-salvation. For the next several months after the discovery of the tumor, every doctor on my team asked me to repeat this story. No matter how many times they heard it, it always rendered them speechless. "This is insane," was the technical assessment of my gynecologist, Dr. Silberstein. She stared wide eyed at me with a continual shake of her head that threatened to continue for days. "You saved your own life," Dr. Kagan concluded. They all wanted to know the same thing: how had I pinpointed the exact location of some cancer hiding inside of me when every single scan had shown nothing?

"I've heard that chemotherapy can bring about psilocybin-like hallucinations," Dr. Menzel had offered when he had his chance to question me. He had listened with rapt attention as I described the months leading up to that surgery. Dr. Menzel had seemed to be the most likely member of the Team of Grownups to accept my visions with unblinking curiosity, so I told him about a few of the things that had happened to me during treatments.

I shrugged. "I have no explanation for whether these were dreams or visions or something else."

Although the doctors seemed happy the tumor was out of me, and they were all fascinated by my self-diagnosis, I still refrained from giving them all the details of what I had seen. In fact, no one except Louis knew the full extent of what I had experienced. It all seemed too crazy. I avoided going into the specifics with anyone else, but especially the doctors. On top of everything, the last thing I needed was for them to think I was losing my mind.

There was no one dream, or specific message focused on the ovary, but the unrelenting stream of dreams for months on end made me better attuned to my body's messages. No voice said, "Hey! You might want to check in your ovary for some cancer, ok?" There was just a nagging feeling that the ovary needed to go. I talked about it so much at home, I think Louis was one step away from buying "Surgery for Dummies" so he could cut it out of me himself.

The follow-up with Dr. Quilici, six months later, would hopefully be the last time I sat in his office until I had my portacath removed. I expected years to pass, not months, before the dreaded thing came out. In the meantime, staying out of his office would be a good sign that my treatments were going well, that there were no new spots on my scan, and that my CEA had stayed where it belonged. All these things together would mean I was holding the recurrence of cancer at bay.

"Remind me again what the name of that ovarian tumor was?" I asked Dr. Quilici. I was sure that he was becoming annoyed with my constant questions about the tumor—six months ago, I had sent him passages from *Round the Twist* to clarify the medical details, and he had specifically named the tumor in his comment window. Although I included the name in the final manuscript, I never thought to commit it to memory.

A little embarrassed, I was asking him yet again to name it. "It's a Krukenberg Tumor. And if we hadn't taken it out, this appointment would have been about something very different." His tone was serious now. He waited for my reaction, the one to confirm the dense mass of his words had finally impacted against my head.

Measuring my facial expression, he spoke again. "You didn't google it, did you?" He angled his head toward me like he was preparing to scold me. After my surgery all those months ago, I mistook his obvious relief at the outcome as a sign that I could pursue all the information I wanted. Turns out his relief was not permission.

I shrugged sheepishly. Without the name of the tumor, I had already stumbled on some scary information when I googled *metastatic colon cancer in an ovary*.

"Don't," he added quickly. He knew there was only a 2.7% chance I was going to follow this advice. He narrowed his eyes at me, probably hoping this trick, which usually bent most people to his will, would work on me. By this point, he knew me better.

I very much appreciated his calm and collected demeanor when discussing this tumor with me. He knows just how devastating cancer treatments are to the body. He saw all my organs with his own eyes—not just the squiggly blobs of a black and white CT scan—and declared that I was disease free. And yet, he could not see the insidious Krukenberg Tumor hiding out in the ovary. I wondered if this would change his recommendations and practices with other young women with colon cancer in the future. In my case, at least, he appeared mildly rattled by the discovery.

Now that I was *technically* disease free, I felt emboldened to do more research on my diagnosis. I had learned more than I ever needed to know about the digestive tract, different cancers and cancer drugs, and even learned how to read the staging classifications in my medical portal notes. But, until this point, I had only been referring to that ovarian tumor as "the last bit of colon cancer" or "that tumor in my ovary" without fully appreciating that this was the thing that would have ultimately killed me.

"You had a time bomb inside of you," Dr. Quilici confirmed. It suddenly became clear just how close to the end of the countdown timer I had come: 3-10 months. These days, I have an actual sense of what life expectancy means. They expected me to be dead during the summer after my diagnosis, this meant I was already nine months into my afterlife. Now I find out my afterlife might have only lasted six months. It really is a heavy burden being a young cancer survivor.

How long was that tiny Krukenberg Tumor hiding out? Had it been there all along, the effects of the chemotherapy and radiation only rendering it unable to grow or spread for a little while? I understood why Dr. Jacobs moved so quickly to begin the adjuvant therapy of Xeloda: to jump on any other metastases that were invisible to the PET or Dr. Quilici's expert eyes, and stunt their growth before they grew out of control, too.

I was now firmly in the phase of cancer treatment that mostly goes unexamined. Flying under the radar, when the primary treatments are finished, they seem to have been successful, yet there are new and ongoing treatments. Everyone, the cancer survivor included, finds out about this stage only when they get to it. I was just as guilty of assuming that once a person has finished chemo and the doctor says, "You're disease free," that it marks the end of the cancer road. I imagined my friends walking out of the doctor's office, doing a celebratory jig on the sidewalk, and then going back to their regular life like nothing ever happened. No one spoke of adjuvant chemotherapies or maintenance drugs or anything like that. They only told me about these things when I found myself at this point.

Ella shared with me that her adjuvant treatments went on for a year after they declared her disease free. She did not speak to anyone about it. She was so desperate for her treatments to be over, for people to stop looking at her with sympathy, that she decided not to talk about what was happening. When I met Ella, she was going through those adjuvant treatments; I was completely unaware of what was happening to her. She was very successful in keeping all of it private. In some ways, I feel as if I let her down—I had not been there to support her the way she had been there for me through my treatments. But now, her ability to protect this part of her life impressed me.

In my case, that ship had already sailed. I was struggling with impressing upon everyone that although treatment continued, it did not mean that the chemotherapy, radiation, or surgeries had been unsuccessful. This was a difficult thing to explain, and I was quickly tiring of it. I had to ask myself: why was it so important that I make every single person understand every single detail of my life? This was an opportunity for me to take a step back. My job was to put the information out there; beyond that, people could do with it whatever they wanted. When people made comments or asked why I was still having treatments, it was ok for me to tell them the facts and let them sort it out.

It seems like very few survivors talk about this part of cancer survival in a public forum. When I mention my adjuvant chemotherapy, commonly, the first reaction of people is to question my doctors' intentions. It is hard enough for them to hear me talk so freely about my cancer and to accept active cancer as part of the conversation. I tried to impart on my friends and family that cancer is not a taboo, we should actually talk about it, and doing so not only helps me move past what happened but also helps them understand the experience better.

But, many had trouble understanding that being declared "disease free" is not the end of the road. Their only point of reference being scenes from television and movies. This made it difficult to explain, so I understood why some felt the need to question my doctors' expertise, or even worse: question *me* and my ability to understand what was happening. Most people had never heard of these treatments. It seems natural they may wonder if my doctor could be wrong or if I might be in denial.

I have been forced to imagine a life without a cure for the cancer that cancer has created in my mind. Few people have considered this is how a survivor might live the rest of their life. So it is easier for them to shut down the conversation at tumors, drugs, and metastases, rather than explore this existential despair. Understandably, this can be too much for most people to bear.

The Krukenberg Tumor was the perfect example of what "Living with Cancer" means. There are expected emotional consequences of having gone through a cancer diagnosis. At the top of my worry list is having to live with the idea of recurrence at some point in my life. I am not alone in this fear. Louis often worries as much as I do about each upcoming scan and expresses his deep concern that the cancer will come back. We are afraid to take my good health for granted, because that is exactly when the rug will get pulled out from under us.

What is harder to explain are the daily fears emanating from in my bones. Did chemo and radiation leave my body at such a deficit that cancer can easily take advantage of me and return within a couple of years? Fun fact: cancer is a side-effect of radiation treatment for cancer. Did I kill one cancer only to cause a new one down the line? I know that every minor ache and pain is not cancer, but it has not stopped me from worrying every time I feel a slight cramp in my belly. Was that more colon cancer or just gas? Usually just gas, but I will never forget that time when it was cancer.

We found the Krukenberg Tumor not because anyone went looking for it or because I was having symptoms, but because I had the sheer dumb luck of pinpointing it myself. Wondering if there are more little tumors hiding out in my body that no one can see scares me. I have never had a scan of my head. Of course, I worry about tumors popping up in my brain; every slight headache scares me. Do I have brain cancer?

I sit here and wonder if Nurse Negative Nancy was right and if I really do only have ten years left—what does that even look like? How would I cope with knowing I have less than ten? What would I stop doing, what would I change, and what would I embrace? It is all too awful to consider. And while I am distracted by these thoughts, will my car cross the center line and kill me, anyway?

I must draw strength from Ella and Alice, both over 10-year cancer survivors, who are living—no, *thriving*—beyond their diagnoses and treatments. We share stories, and I can cry on their shoulders whenever I need to, but the message they transmit to me is the same: just live.

Vicky

I am always the center of attention. Nearly every social situation can be bent to my will. When I was in college, I somehow organized everyone in my year into a troupe, the camaraderie exceeding what anyone remembered happening in previous years. Our class probably was one of the most unified and socially connected that had ever passed through those halls. I liked to think I played a role in that. Louis brings me to client dinners and industry parties, and I end up as the one being asked questions about my life. Louis calls it charm. I know no other way to be.

It would only be a matter of time before I bent the Disney Family Cancer Center (DFCC) patients and doctors to my will. Louis saw it coming based on the way I had drawn the nurses to me during my hospital stay after my colectomy and diagnosis. At my first appointments at Dr. Jacobs' office, I was unsure of what I was getting in to. I was timid at the reception desk; I was nervous with the nurses. Yet I found a way to just be myself in the way Louis says is hypnotizing. Within just a few weeks, one nurse told me that when my name is on the daily schedule, the nurses vie over who gets to draw my blood.

In only a few visits, I took over the infusion center as well. Even feeling shitty while I was getting my chemotherapy, I drew people to me. I have some sort of gravity that no one escapes. Nurses not involved in my care would visit with me. Terry and Abby, my infusion nurses, were showing the other nurses my portal profile picture (a dynamic black-and-white photo of me doing crow pose, an impressive yoga arm balance), and those nurses wanted to see me for themselves. When I was getting hydration during the last week of my radiation treatments, the nurses took turns for the opportunity to give it to me. I was like some strange cancer celebrity, and I did not even feel 100% like myself. They had no idea what they were in for once I felt better.

When I began my Avastin treatments in January, it felt great to talk with Abby without the haze of drugs clouding my brain. And just like at parties, I was the life of the infusion center. Leaving my curtain open meant that every nurse in the ward would come by to say hello, and for whatever reason, other patients, virtual strangers, waved to me as they walked through the common area to choose their cubicle for the day.

At the start of those treatments, I was overflowing with positivity and enthusiasm. I was not sitting in the waiting room looking crumpled and struggling to hold my head up. I knew where to go, what to do, who to speak to. I had all the confidence that comes with experience and familiarity. I was now one of those people who the nurses at the front desk greeted by name. I was someone who had been around the ward a few times. And then someone appeared who had an even deeper familiarity with the 4th Floor Oncology Department: Vicky.

One morning, as I waited for my appointment with Dr. Jacobs, the elevator doors in the waiting room opened like stage curtains and an older couple made their grand entrance into my life—the husband pushing his wife in a wheelchair. Their conversation was lively, despite her outward exhaustion from treatments, and immediately Louis and I were smitten with their charm.

"Is there someone back there?" the woman asked her husband as he pushed her up to the desk. Her head well below the counter, she could not see the nurse beyond the window.

"Yes, and she's very beautiful," he answered her. I heard Louis chuckle next to me; I could not take my eyes off of these two lovebirds.

While they were still engaged in their friendly banter with the nurse, I was called in to Dr. Jacobs' office. "How charming were they?" Louis said as I stepped up on the scale. My weight was still stuck on the same number as the day I finished radiation five months earlier. I admit, I was not eating excessive amounts, but I was not limiting my intake, either. Dr. Jacobs and the nurses continued to tell me that worrying about it would only make gaining weight more difficult.

After my physical and blood draw, we returned to the infusion center's half of the waiting area to find the older couple also there. I checked in at the desk and got my hospital wristband, while Louis sat down. And then the conversation shifted into high gear. I could hear Louis, who rarely engages with strangers the way I do, laughing, and the couple chattering away with him. "That's my wife, Lisa," I heard him say, so I turned around and gave a friendly wave.

By the time I finished signing in and could join the party, Louis, Gary, and Vicky were old friends. The conversation turned to our glasses, which were always fogging up because of the surgical masks; I gave them a handful of the anti-fog masks I carried in my day bag. I thought nothing of it—I have a giant box of masks at home and Gary's glasses were fogging now. It seemed the obvious thing to do. We wished them good luck when I was called into the infusion center.

A few minutes later, getting comfortable in my favorite corner cubicle, our new friend Gary appeared around my curtain. He was "pretend" sheepish because, clearly, he was not shy. Not being shy either, I know that game—I often have to play it when I am not familiar with someone and am trying not to overwhelm them with my friendliness—and so I appreciated his manner.

"My wife, Vicky, wanted me to give you this," he said, handing me a sheet of purple stationery with their handwritten contact information on it. "We hope you'll stay in touch with us."

"Absolutely!" I said, happily taking the paper.

The simple act of giving them the new masks made them want to know us better.

My infusion of Avastin is supposed to take only 20 minutes. Most days, it takes longer than that for the lab to analyze my blood tests before the pharmacist sends out my drugs. On this day, I used the hour-long break between blood draw and portacath puncture to stretch my legs and use the restroom. I wanted to say one more hello to the couple before she started her drugs. I saw Gary, returning from the water cooler, slip through the curtain of a familiar cubicle—it was the same one that Suzy always chose. Although this smaller room faces east, the sun somehow mysteriously seems to avoid it, giving it the feel of a cozy cave. I thought it was an endearing coincidence that Vicky's favorite cubicle was also Suzy's. My heart smiled.

Vicky had already beaten breast cancer over a decade ago but was now going through several chemotherapy treatments to curtail the latest metastasis in her lungs. Every few months, they changed her drug combination—some she would no longer get, while new ones, especially immunotherapies, were added. When I met her today, she was still getting the heavy stuff; I got a glimpse of several UV chemo bags hanging from her tree and decided not to bother her.

As soon as I returned to my cubicle, though, I took out my iPhone, entered their contact information, and started typing an email with my thumbs. I did not expect her to respond to me for several days. Vicky's chemotherapy was so serious she needed to ride in and out of the cancer center in a wheelchair. I imagined it would be days before she even thought about looking at a computer screen. Louis and I vowed if we did not hear from them by the weekend, I would pick up the phone and call. This is a big deal. I hate talking on the phone. In fact, most of my friends know the likelihood of me picking up when they call is slim to none.

I did not have to wait even 24 hours before a reply email from Vicky appeared in my inbox. I was over the moon. A new friend, all because of cancer. I wanted to hate cancer so much, and yet, the new friends I have met because of it, Alice, Suzy and now Vicky, made it difficult to resent it.

Once I met Vicky, the infusion center truly became a Social Club. Gary has the same effortless charm that I have moving through life. Vicky said she admired me because I "lived in a world with no strangers." She said this was why so many people were drawn to my energy.

It always delighted us that know our treatments were on the same schedule rotation. Week after week, walking into the infusion center, the first thing I did was look for the cubicle where Gary and Vicky sat, their curtain usually wide open. When Vicky was doing well with her chemo, she joined in on the socializing. Their friendly waves and hellos reaching me clearly through the otherwise silent ward. Vicky was struggling with mobility, so I would visit with her in her cubicle while I waited for the pharmacist to send out my drug. Month after month, all four of us hugged like we were family.

Vicky was fighting her third occurrence of cancer—she was in a much more weakened physical state than I was. At this point, I was *technically* disease free. Yet, these two were more worried about how I was feeling. I would ask Vicky, "How are you?" Her answers were always short, "I'm surviving," followed by, "But how are you, sweetheart?" She never allowed the conversation to dwell on herself. I was always touched.

Once her infusions started, though, I would hug them both one more time and go back to my cubicle, waiting for the nurses to arrive with my medication. Often, Gary would make his way back to my room to stand and talk with Louis and me while Vicky napped through her infusion. The nurses bustled around all of us, seemingly unbothered by our socializing in the small cubicles—even though it made their job more difficult.

We always visited during our infusions, Gary and I making trips back and forth between the cubicles to sit and chat. I realized we were the only people doing any visiting. The nurses were caught up in our activity, but the other patients were silent. I felt too alive to be silent—and so did Vicky. She was going to fight this thing until the end. Cancer would not make her shrink and hide; she was visiting friends, going places, and living her life. Which was more than I was doing at that point. I was still nervous about going to the store, running errands, and attending my first orchestra rehearsal. Vicky was an inspiration for how to live with grace and joy. Compared to her, I was failing miserably; I had no excuse for my paralysis.

Gary made an offhanded comment to me about how I reminded him of Vicky so much, and it was no wonder we had all become friends. I really hoped we could see them outside of the cancer center sometime soon. We could all use some time together without the shadow of cancer blocking our view of the sun.

My infusion complete, I needed to make one more visit with Vicky before we left. "We just love you both so much," Vicky said, hugging Louis. When it was my turn, I held on to her and told her I loved her fiercely. It was always difficult to walk away from her. My heart ached. Vicky was going to spend the next few days reeling from her chemotherapy, and there was nothing I could do to soothe her.

We were silent in the elevator ride to the bottom floor. Louis knew I was thinking of Vicky and kept reminding me she was strong and still fighting. The front doors slid open, and we stepped out into the sunlight. Without breaking stride, someone crashed straight into me—Suzy wrapped me up in a hug that never seemed to want to end. Just when my heart was breaking with a goodbye, I was gifted this intense hello.

I have felt nothing like the hugs Suzy and I share—like we are combining our powers. If we were witches, we would be a powerful coven. We had a way of combining our magic, infusing the other with strength and positivity. And never sucking the life force from the other.

Today, Dr. Jacobs had called her in to discuss her next treatment plan—things were not going in the right direction. She had already had six doses each, of FOLFOXIRI and FOLFIRI chemotherapies. She was supposed to have her sigmoid colon removed, the source of her cancer. The surgery was scheduled; she had completed the pre-op scans, X-rays, blood tests, and physical. Removing this part of the colon would not only eliminate the physical source of the disease but also provide emotional relief from carrying around the affected intestine. For the first time in a long time, she was full of hope and positivity, knowing that this part of her suffering would soon have a resolution.

Unfortunately, her pre-op PET scan had revealed the unexpected: a glowing spot near her spine indicating hypermetabolic activity. Although this explained the persistent back pain she had been having for several months, it was far from good news. There was no hoping this was just a slipped disc or arthritis. This little light on the scan signaled the beginning of yet another leg in the race for her life. Would there be a third round of chemo? Would she have to have radiation this time? How would this affect the upcoming surgery? The best we could hope was that her body had healed enough in the past six months for her to endure the onslaught of treatments looming on her horizon.

She looked wonderful, though. Unlike me, she had not lost her hair with all that chemo. Full of life and energy, she was sporting a new layer of fat in her cheeks, and I no longer felt her shoulder blades under my hands as we hugged. She was vibrant, healthy, and youthful. I hoped she could maintain this vigor during the next stage.

In the meantime, she was spending as much time with her family as she could. Her son was fast approaching 7 years old, and she was keeping up with him. The family was planning a trip to South Korea to visit relatives. This was a good sign. I hoped the new treatments would not start right away, giving her a few extra weeks of normalcy before being knocked down again.

My own fortunate situation felt more precarious after hearing Suzy's news. I felt great. Despite my lack of success in getting back into my life, I had loads of energy. But I was like that two years ago, before cancer. There was no hint that cancer was eating away at my intestine—little did I know I was about to face the greatest challenge of my life. This left me with a residual disbelief and distrust of my own body. Was there something inside of me regrowing, hiding, biding its time, waiting for another lull in my energy to take over and try to kill me again? If a new mass could grow inside of Suzy after twelve doses of chemo, could the same happen to me? I only had six doses. Would my next scan in April be the one that revealed a new tumor inside of me, too?

It is difficult to trust again after cancer. Before, I took so much for granted. I went to bed every night assuming I would wake up the next morning; I drove my car on the freeway, never questioning whether I would make it to my destination without an accident. And worst of all, even as I was going through the diagnosis process, holding the PET scan that told the clear tale of stage-4 metastatic cancer, I still never questioned whether I would be alive the following week to enjoy Thanksgiving dinner with all our boys. Even faced with hard facts, I never stopped to consider it could all end in the blink of an eye. That is how out-of-touch I was with my mortality.

Now, everything seems more treacherous, whether that is a simple cough—*do I have lung cancer?*—or stiffness in my back—*do I have spine cancer?*—or a pain in my hand—*do I have hand cancer?* Will a simple cold turn into pneumonia? Is that pain in my gut a new tumor? I worry every time Andrew gets in the car—I worry about people running red lights or turning left in front of him. When I hear sirens blaring from the nearby firehouse, I worry about a fire in our attic—do we really know what is going on with the electrical wiring up there?

Should I reconsider going to orchestra rehearsals again, knowing most people are choosing not to wear masks anymore? Everyone seems so accustomed to living in a world with COVID-19 that they are numb and ambivalent to the risk. With my very low white blood cell count, and lack of booster vaccines, any exposure to the coronavirus could spiral out of control faster than I could fight it off. Would I survive cancer, rush back to rehearsals because I am impatient, only to be killed by COVID? I feared I was on a knife's edge between normal-level concerns and clinical psychosis.

If I lived my life consumed with a fear of COVID, cancer, common colds, and traffic accidents, I would never leave the house. Was it better to be healthy but safely locked away? Or to go out and live, taking my chances with accidents and germs? Even though the answer was obvious, I was still cowering behind my front door.

I read on the patio, watched the hummingbirds fight over the feeders, and enjoyed the unseasonably warm afternoons. I also visited with the once familiar ghosts of my previous life. After all this time, I was used to being a delicate cancer patient quarantining inside my home; how could I just jump back into my life as if none of this mattered?

Close to a dozen small birds have gotten into our house this year. They slip in through the open patio door when the dogs push it open to let themselves out. Most of these wayward birds find their way out the same way they came in. But one morning, a small bird flew in and took a trip through the house, focusing its escape efforts on the picture window in the formal living room where our pianos live. The telltale sound of a bird hitting itself against the glass led me straight to it. When I found the little bird, it was resting on the windowsill, staring out at freedom beyond its invisible prison bars. I had to act fast before the dogs realized what was happening.

"Sh…" I cooed, getting as close as I could. For whatever reason, I am an expert at catching birds. Maybe because I had a parakeet when I was a kid or because I have placed a lot of baby birds back in their nests, I have an innate ability to get birds to trust me. When one gets trapped inside our house, I take advantage of this superpower and always get them back outside with as little stress as possible.

I held my finger out toward the bird. It must have been inside the house for quite some time, because it was exhausted. It gave a quick glance at my finger. For a moment, I thought it might hop onto it and I would simply walk to the back door and set it free. It turned away from my hand, shunning me like it was considering the other rescue options. There were none. "Ok, ok, sh sh sh…" I kept repeating. I made a few little kissy noises, hoping that would somehow convince it to trust me. This bird was exhausted and ready to give up. Time for Plan B.

Carefully, I cupped my hands and gently closed them around the little bird. I felt its nails trying to find a grip on my palm, its beak pressing into my finger. Quickly, I rushed to the backdoor—I would not hold it any longer than necessary. On the patio, I opened my hands, expecting the bird to fly off instantly. But it waited. It hopped onto the finger I had originally offered and perched there for a moment. It looked around the yard, perhaps deciding where it was going to go, perhaps confused by the sudden change of scenery, or perhaps paralyzed by its brush with a human.

Whatever its reason, I marveled at its weight on my finger, how strong its tiny nails dug into my skin, and how perfectly comfortable it had made itself on its new perch. "Good luck," I said to it. I know it didn't understand me. But for a brief second, it turned its head and looked straight at me. Then, with the slightest push, it became weightless and flew off into the trees.

In this year since Dr. Jacobs declared, "No visible sign of disease," I have been fluttering around aimlessly inside the house, bouncing off the windows. My exit route was clear, open, and waiting for me to walk through it. I would see it if I just stopped bouncing off the glass.

A Weighty Subject

I grew up in the 1980s, the decade of fluorescent jelly shoes, Aquanet hairspray, over the top materialism, and unrealistic body images. Our moms were working out to television exercise shows like Richard Simmons', stocking up on Jane Fonda videocassette tapes, and buying ThighMasters to use while they watched *Dynasty* after the kids went to bed. Teenagers were trying every diet craze that came along, popping Dexatrim pills, and barfing in the girls' bathroom after lunch. My mother was not immune to the expectations either. Every morning, she would stand, in her underwear, on the bathroom scale and bemoan whatever number it was that she saw. I never knew the exact number, but I am certain it was not very high. She just thought she was supposed to weigh less—three pounds less, to be exact.

As a teenage girl, I was bombarded with images of the body type I was expected to have thanks to Teen Beat Magazine, Kate Moss, MTV videos, Calvin Klein and Benetton ads, and the struggles of Tracey Gold. I knew I was supposed to be skinny, because the magazines said that was what boys wanted. When I was in high school, I went through a phase where I tried not eating. But that lasted exactly until dinner time; I was hungry, and I had no willpower to starve. While other girls were working on their own unrealistic goals by drinking Slim Fast shakes, I questioned my commitment to meeting the expectations. I was active—on the Varsity Swim Team and ran 2 miles every morning before school with my brother—I was healthy and strong. In reality, I had nothing to worry about, even if I did not look like the girls in the magazines.

I was one of the smallest kids in class and shorter than all my friends in elementary school. At that age, I hardly even noticed. It only bothered me when I reached 6th grade and noticed the other girls were wearing training bras while I was still standing on the books at the bottom of my locker to reach the ones on the top shelf. I would not reach 5-feet tall until I was 13 years old; another year passed before I was wearing bras and getting my first period. My final towering height of 5-foot 3-inches resulted from a growth spurt before college.

As a young adult, I learned how to bend my small stature to my advantage. For almost a decade after I graduated from college, I found work as a decoy musician in college orchestras around New England. I looked young, and being short, I was not easily visible from the audience's perspective. Several times each year, colleges throughout the region hired me to play in their orchestra when they did not have oboe students enrolled. On the flip side, this same characteristic made it difficult for me to be taken seriously in my first collegiate teaching job. When I walked into the music office at the state college to pick up my office key at the start of my first semester on the job, the office staff thought I was a student and would not give it to me. The Dean of Music stepped in to explain who I was. It was embarrassing for all involved. Three decades later, I think fondly on the days when I could still be mistaken for a college student.

Thanks to fitness, I never actually struggled with my weight. I had a rock-solid weight because I had a daily exercise routine alternating between yoga and running. I was active, vegan, and as healthy as a young woman could be. These healthy habits have stayed with me my whole life, and because of that, I could always count on my weight being steady within a tiny, five-pound window.

The rare times my weight plummeted unexpectedly were always tied to some sort of emotional issue. During my divorce, I dropped an unexpected 10 pounds. My doctor chalked it up to depression. He was right—once I got that under control, my weight came right back up. When my weight dropped in the months ahead of my cancer diagnosis, I assumed it was depression again. The COVID pandemic had left me unemployed, making this a reasonable explanation, at least for the first five pounds.

In *Round the Twist,* I avoided using specific numbers when talking about my weight. I spoke in broad strokes, the details of that weight loss given as how much I lost without the specific number of where I started. I decided that in this book, I would need to talk specifics. I can only fully explain the mind games of weight loss without ambiguities. Numbers make this a lot easier to deal with and less confusing for you, Dear Reader.

At 5 feet 3 inches tall, my normal weight is 120 pounds—well within the expected healthy weight spectrum. Despite all my healthy habits, I still inherited my mother's desire to see that number go lower. Regardless of how many miles I ran, how much yoga I did, or how little I ate, this number was always difficult to bring down. Of course, sometimes the number crept up. This happened whenever I was pulled out of my normal routines, most recently when Louis and I were buying this house and eating takeout more than usual. The stress relieved as we settled into the new house, the scale slid happily back to 120.

In the first year of the COVID pandemic, I put on a little weight. We were ordering delivery more often, and I was boredom snacking. With the State Park closed, I was not meeting my weekly hiking and running quota. My concert clothes were a little snug at my first concert after the lockdown ended. Not wanting to spend money on a new concert wardrobe, I resolved to lose those new pounds. No more Thai food delivery every Friday. It was time to buckle down and get back on track. By the end of that summer, I was losing weight. At first, I was relieved. That enthusiasm distracted me from noticing that it was happening at a faster than normal rate.

I hate getting weighed at the doctor's office. No matter how fancy my scale is at home (we have one of those new-fangled digital ones that, if you stand on it long enough, will show your body fat percentage among other statistics), the doctor's office scale is always higher by 2 pounds. At every doctor appointment, I have to do the office-to-home conversion.

In the spring of 2021, the COVID lockdown had just crossed the one-year mark, and I had spent that year not caring about what I ate. I was tired of the lockdown; I was frustrated from not working; I was eating to soothe my annoyance. Losing weight was secondary at this point—I could worry about my weight at some mystical day in the future when the lockdown ended.

When I stepped on the scale at my gynecologist's office in August 2021, the scale read 128—no wonder my concert clothes were a little snug last month. "Ok, just remember, it's really 126 at home," I convinced myself, trying to stay cool knowing the nurse does not write down the number I have in my head—she takes the one from the scale. Next time, I would remember to face away from the weights and balances. My food fueled pandemic would have to end. I would need to up my running mileage and lower my calories. This weight was not empirically unhealthy or a problem. I just wanted to see 120 again, and be done with it. If I did the work, then I could lose this lockdown weight.

There was no way of knowing I would spend the next three months going through the diagnosis process. Cancer consumed all the calories I was taking in; pounds were falling off of me. Week after week, the scale at the doctor's office would show another two pounds lost. My primary physician, Dr. Kagan, was concerned with my weight loss, but I was pleased to lose those pandemic pounds, plus a little extra—I was a few pounds under my normal weight. This made yoga a little easier, and my jeans fit better. Who could complain?

Meanwhile the first oncologist I saw, Dr. Messina[2], who I fired after only two office visits, never even acknowledged the weight loss, despite having all my medical records and notes from Dr. Kagan. While the first team of doctors blew me off, I was withering away. My extremely low weight disturbed Louis; he spent much of his time trying to feed me. Even with the increased calories, I was still losing. We had now reached the point where our spider senses were tingling. Something was wrong, and no one was listening to us.

Weight loss is a huge red flag leading up to a cancer diagnosis. Cancer is ravenously greedy. It steals whatever calories go into the body for itself. After my colectomy and five days of recovery in the hospital, I was down to 108. I think the last time I weighed that, I was in 9th grade. I had lost 18 pounds in fourteen weeks. I looked fragile and unbalanced. My clothes were hanging off me, and I was very much afraid.

"None of this will work if she doesn't eat," had been Dr. Quilici's very important advice. In the four weeks between my surgery and the start of chemo, Louis worked very hard, overfeeding me every day in an attempt to put some weight on me. I managed to put back four precious pounds, and Dr. Jacobs declared I should aim to stay within five pounds of this, in either direction, during chemotherapy. It was difficult, but I worked hard to maintain my weight. Thanks to Louis' tireless efforts to make me eat, even when I had no appetite, we kept my weight within Dr. Jacobs' prescribed range.

Fat is something our body actually needs. Without it, we lack nutritional reserves and the obvious insulation. Even though it was late spring, I was chilled most of the time. I wore sweaters

---

[2] Although Dr. Messina is a real doctor, the name has been changed.

and long sleeves while everyone else was breaking out their T-shirts. I never considered the importance of fat before I had none.

After chemo, I had twelve weeks to focus on my weight before radiation treatments began, and I think I did a bang-up job! My weight at home was up to 119 pounds, but I still looked thin; cancer had forced my body to use up its fat reserves before resorting to consuming muscle. My butt cheeks were absolutely flattened, and my breasts were at least one cup size smaller. But I was alive, and now my body was happily storing some much-needed fat during this downtime. Radiation put the new pounds to work. No one on my oncology team was concerned about my limited diet of noodles. My nutritionist kept repeating, "Calories are calories. We don't care what you eat, just eat."

After a week of hydration, my radiation oncology nurse, Cindy, had me hop on the scale. "You've had six days of IV fluids. You're going to be amazed at what that does to your weight!" She giggled as I stepped on the office scale—the LED screen blinked 121. "Don't worry, I'm not writing this in your chart," she smiled. This *was* hilarious. We giggled like teenagers on the way to the exam room. The IV fluids, 2 liters every day, added up the pounds. Thankfully, those "fake pounds" would make all the difference for my immediate recovery. My body would slowly give up that water weight during the next five days, so that when I stepped on the scale for my follow-up appointment with Dr. Jacobs, we all saw my new doctor's office weight: 112.6.

I would stay at that number for the next seven months. No matter what I did, no matter how much I ate, or how much junk food I stuffed into my face, the scale was stuck at 112.6. I was enjoying this freedom of consumption, but also worrying about why it was so difficult to gain. Both Dr. Jacobs and Dr. Kagan would continually remind me, "This is just what you weigh now. Your body has been through quite an ordeal." Obviously, they were right. My body was more interested in using the calories to heal itself, not to store fat. I was also missing 8 inches of intestine after my colostomy reversal surgery, and my body needed to close those wounds. I focused on eating healthy, exercising to gain muscle, and trying not to stress about things that were out of my control.

Shopping was difficult. When I found something cute to try on, there was a low likelihood there was an XS or size-0 on the rack. And even if they had the size, the XS shirts were overhanging my shoulders. I looked like I was playing dress-up in my big sister's closet. Frustrated and deflated when salespeople suggested I shop online for petite sizes—or worse, go to the junior-miss section—I felt isolated among the racks of pretty clothes I would not be buying. Standing at a mirror in the middle of Macy's, draped in an oversized-extra-small blazer, I wanted to say to every person who passed me by, "See? This is what cancer does to you." The only item of clothing that always fits better with weight loss is jeans, so purchasing new jeans that fit properly made me feel a little better and helped me embrace my new thinner body.

Despite wanting to lose weight for years, I never expected to dislike weighing so little. Here I was at the very bottom of the weight range for my height, and it was painfully obvious. My friends said, "You look great, but you're so thin." This is not actually a compliment. It would be important to get up to 114 on my home scale. My nurses implied that gaining back all the weight I lost might be impossible after cancer.

What I did not expect was that when the scale began creeping up toward that new goal weight of 114, I would resist it mightily. I felt just as weird about putting on important recovery weight as I did about gaining those 6 pounds during the pandemic: not good.

We women really do a number on ourselves with body image. That number on the scale is never right, no matter how low it gets. I wondered if when I hit my goal weight, I would again pine for a lower weight. My mother did not stand a chance, and, although it was not her intention—I am certain she never thought that I was watching and absorbing her body image issues for myself—she passed on these insecurities that would haunt me through my cancer treatments and beyond.

The trick was to be thankful for every pound I gained back. I had to learn to celebrate my recovery and survival. When the scale finally flashed 114, I had to remind myself to be happy about it. Holding on to weight was an obvious side effect of improving health. Though I had only gained two pounds this year, everyone was telling me I looked healthy. For whatever reason, I still made a point of saying, "I've only gained two pounds."

I learned that there was a pronounced difference between a sickly 115 during cancer treatments and a healthy 115 after cancer. My face was filling out, my thighs were looking a little curvier, and my posture was getting better. I looked and felt healthy. I just needed my mind to catch up and accept this little bit of weight gain as necessary. Flipping my attitude on its head after decades of wanting to lose weight was a monumental effort. It was a heavy emotional lift to accept this sign that I was firmly on the road to recovery.

Chasing Smoke

It started with a simple idea: I am going to get back to work. Work meant getting back on stage and performing again. A little over a year ago, I was careening toward cancer's cliff, my career slipping through my fingers, grasping desperately on to my cello bow. Through the pain and fear, music was a lifeline to normalcy. If I was working and distracted, then I could not be sick. I convinced myself that everything was ok because I was sitting on stage.

As the weeks pressed on, I backed out of concerts, canceled on commitments, and walked out of rehearsals. The pain was overtaking my life. Perhaps I was being naïve because I believed I would just be taking a break. Maybe a few weeks, or a month, if I needed surgery. I assumed the pain was from the giant ovarian cysts that were growing out of control. It was time to be done with endometriosis, something I had been dealing with since I was a teenager. I thought I would have a hysterectomy, be in the hospital for a few days, followed by a couple of weeks of recovery. Before I knew it, I would be well enough for the winter holiday concerts.

Never once did I dream it would be colon cancer, or that my career would go on pause for a year and a half. It would have seemed an outrageous outcome. Even faced with the serious bowel blockage, I believed I would have the swollen part of my colon taken out and a new diet to follow. I would play *The Nutcracker* in December like nothing happened. Even while staring down the barrel of a cancer diagnosis, my brain fought it every step of the way.

But then I was handed a death sentence with an unknown execution date. Now facing an uncertain future, living became my only goal; getting back on stage was pushed to the second page of my to-do list. The cello could wait. I only had one job now: survival.

Chemotherapy, radiation, and several surgeries well behind me, I was on my way to good health at a speed I could not control, dragging my feet through the dirt like a little kid trying to stop a bike without brakes. Since I was feeling so well, I said yes to playing a concert in March. Having given up the holiday concert just a couple months before this, I had time to mentally prepare myself for the next performance on the schedule. My colleagues were delighted to hear I was coming back. But, underneath my bravado, I was hiding the truth: I was terrified. Thinking about the upcoming first rehearsal, I regretted agreeing to play at all.

I just needed more time. More time to practice. More time to build my calluses back. More time to grow my hair. More time to try leaving the house. I felt stressed whenever Louis and I went anywhere besides the hospital or cancer center or the doctors' offices. For a year, I had been neatly tucked away at home, in a safe little bubble where there was nothing to worry about except surviving cancer. A place where there were no major decisions to be made other than what bland food I might eat for dinner or what Netflix series we would binge-watch. It was a cozy existence where pants were optional, there was no need to cover my chemo curls, and I could wear slippers on the back patio.

What do people wear to the grocery store? Do women really put on makeup before going out? Was it ok to wear jeans when we went out to lunch? What shoes did I used to wear with my brown corduroys? Sometimes I forgot what shirts I had hanging in the back of the closet; looking through my clothes felt like a day at the mall—every outfit was new and exciting.

Having not interacted with anyone in person except my medical team for the past year, I worried that I might have forgotten how to function in polite society. Would I remember how to order a coffee at Starbucks? Would I remember how to play in tune if I went to a rehearsal? And would I remember to turn on the headlights when I drove home? The routines that everyone takes for granted felt like brand new requirements for me. I was a toddler unleashed in a tea house.

My stomach lurched when Suzy invited me to lunch. She simply said, "We should go to lunch sometime soon." *Soon* could mean anything. Besides, she might cancel on me because of a sudden pain too severe to leave the house. With the dark cloud of cancer-induced social anxiety hanging over me, I found comfort in knowing it was just as likely she would cancel at the last minute as I would. I hoped since she was going through the same as me, it meant she had made the invitation with no expectations attached. Of course, I was making a lot of assumptions about her, since she had already been doing more outside her house than I had. Projecting my own fears on to her only gave me an excuse to cancel on her first.

Ella mentioned she would like to bring food to my house so we could spend an afternoon together. We had not seen each other for a few months—she had her own health issues to deal with. But now everyone was healthy and ready to mingle. I was looking forward to scheduling our next lunch date until the email arrived in my inbox. "I'll pick up lunch and bring it over any day you want," she offered. I thought I would collapse with fear—just reading the words made the butterflies in my stomach take flight. *Remember, this is just a suggestion*, I told myself. She would never show up at my door unannounced.

Thankfully, Ella understood what I was going through, having been through it herself. Rejoining the real world after her cancer over a decade ago had been a complicated process. But to the rest of us, she had appeared brave, jumping into life with both feet. I met her during her recovery period, and I remember nothing that betrayed what was going on inside of her.

But I could not hide forever. I would have to get back to real life. What would that look like? Despite what some of my stranger social ticks may imply, I am not shy. *Round the Twist* was creeping closer to its publication date, and I was finding my footing with marketing and advertising. I had a shiny new website and plastered an enormous picture of my face beside an "About the Author" caption. Because my eyes continued to be plagued with infections after chemotherapy, I toyed with retaking the photo because the sty in my left eye seemed hugely obvious and distracting. Louis reassured me I could see it only because I knew it was there; no one else would notice it. He also said the new lines by my eyes and the grey hairs that cancer had given me made me look professional and wise. I usually trust his opinion, so I figured he was on to something. The photo made me look like I might know what I was doing with this book thing. "Slap a pair of glasses on my face, twist a scarf around my neck, and suddenly I look like a writer!" I joked, suggesting this should be my author biography.

I was excited about promoting the book. The thought of traveling around the country to wellness centers, support groups, conferences, and book launch events was thrilling. I enjoyed posting updates to my social media, announcing web interviews and travel dates. Why was I excited about book events but not orchestra rehearsals?

The book made me feel brave. It made me feel like I had a purpose. When I walked into a room, people wanted to hear what I had to say. I was no expert on cancer, but I was an expert on my story. The infusion staff, doctors, nurses—everyone—told me I had "a great attitude" during my treatments. The book allowed me the rare gift of viewing myself objectively. During the editing process, I read my book ad nauseam for four months and an amazing thing happened: I met myself. And *Lisa in the Book* was someone I could relate to. She was snarky, upbeat, and sometimes inspiring. Although it was difficult to reread the emotional parts, the book left me with an overwhelming sense of hope and joy. Maybe the book could do the same for other people.

The United Ostomy Association of America was holding its annual conference in Houston, and I had registered to set up a display to sell my book there. I parked myself behind a table with 25 copies, and engaged with other ostomates. Quickly, I learned how to talk about myself as a character in a book. The more I talked, the more I understood what the book was about. The book's message was a positive one—bringing hope to other cancer patients. It was fun to travel by myself; the solo adventure allowed me to glimpse the amazing things that might happen if I were brave enough to turn the page on this new chapter of my life. What would be the title of this new chapter?

Lisa the Musician had not accomplished half the goals she set as a bright-eyed and bushy-tailed college graduate. I am proud of my accomplishments as a teacher, having made my mark on the impressionable youth from coast to coast. But what about my performing career? I had spent every day since I was 4 years old playing an instrument, envisioning myself on a stage in an orchestra making music. I had taken several orchestral auditions in the first few years following college graduation. Although I was full of confidence and energy, I won only one of them, and it happened to be the very first one. It was for a substitute position in a small orchestra, the pay barely covered the cost of gas to make the four-hour round trip to the city in the next state. I had devoted my whole life to learning and performing music. Twenty-five years after that first audition win, where was I now? Why was I wasting so much time practicing when there was nothing to practice for? I was becoming disillusioned. Was this what I wanted to focus on in the second half of my life?

Without a well-paying job or clear career path stretched out in front of me, why was I so determined to keep on this trajectory? I worked so hard into my 30s to reach a reasonable peak. But from there it was just a steady roll backward down the hill. Just before my diagnosis, I was mostly volunteering my time and talents, and I was losing interest in pursuing something more involved. I lacked the motivation to take auditions. The probability of brilliant success was going down with each passing concert season.

The community orchestras I played with would be there, no matter what else I was doing in my life. I could go back any time I wanted. But would I ever be ready? That I was feeling anxiety and ambivalence over returning should have been a big red flag. Most of my college friends have either landed big jobs in orchestras or universities or have moved on to another non-music career, while my teeth were clamped on useless scraps. Constantly changing goals and direction, I was used to restarting and recreating my career. Without a full-time orchestra job, I freelanced. Not enough freelance work? I can teach private lessons. If I am not teaching enough kids, then I will... fill in the blanks. I was chasing smoke.

The book made me question my narrow view of music as my only talent and career option—might there be something else I could do with my life? The book was unique. Just the mere mention of the book started opening doors for me. It was like there was a bright light shining on it. I was not the only person in their 40s who had gone through this horrendous experience of cancer. I did it with smiles and laughter, outshining the sadness and pain. If I could do it, then maybe I could help someone else do it.

I would continue to practice my cello and decided that I would join in on rehearsals and concerts when I felt like it. My life was about to be scheduled around book events, support groups, and conferences. There is a purpose. There is hope. I could put my natural charm and ability to lead to good use. This was not about ego. This was about a clear path laid out before me, paved in my strongest attributes. Would I be brave enough to step on to it? Or would I stand there on the threshold, paralyzed by a little voice whispering, "You really shouldn't." Fear would be the first to greet me. Would I be brave enough to push past?

I had started over many times in my life: changing what instrument I play, picking up the pieces of my heart after a divorce, moving across the country. I have reinvented myself continuously throughout my life. I have never been just "one thing." I am someone who has viewed each new obstacle as an opportunity to grow. Perhaps this is not about choosing between being a musician or a writer, but about finding the things that bring me joy. It is time to stop labeling myself as one thing only and jamming myself into a predetermined category. Maybe I am not the square peg; maybe I am the box with all the different shaped holes cut into it.

Since I was a child, I have instinctually known how to talk to people and charm them into listening. And that has followed me into adulthood. My identity has always been wrapped up in performing, speaking, or making up silly dances. Pam has pointed out that I never just stand around and talk to colleagues during rehearsals—I hold court. I know she is right. I am the center of attention when I speak. People form a circle around me. My whole life, I have had this power. It was time to put it to good use.

I imagined myself standing in front of an audience, reading excerpts from my book, answering questions, and maybe even signing books. My signature in their copy would give them a piece of the experience to hold on to—a memento of our connection. A fleeting word, a singular sentence, might make a difference in someone's life. I never liked the platitude "Everything happens for a reason." Instead, I asked myself, "For what purpose will I use this experience?" The answer was presenting itself with every imaginary swoop of my future blue ink pen.

And while I was exploring my new horizons, I was anxious about the upcoming rehearsal in ten days that would mark my return to the stage. I had a million excuses for why I should back out of the concert: there would not be enough room on the small stage for me; my wrists hurt; and my bowels were not 100% potty trained to get through a 4-hour stretch. It would be easy to get out of this thing. As the days ticked down, I made my plans to call to the conductor. I could tell him the truth, and he would understand because he had been a part of my support circle. In the end, none of my anxieties mattered. The decision was out of my hands.

Two weeks before the first rehearsal, I scraped my hand on something. Avastin has a bleeding risk, much like blood thinners. These days, a spattering of bruises covered my knees and the backs of my arms thanks to my yoga practice; whenever I bumped my shin or elbow on anything, a new bruise would bloom almost immediately. My gums bled when I brushed my teeth; when I blew my nose, the Kleenexes were filled with blood. For days, the scrape on the back of my hand was red and angry. There was a bullseye on it—I was constantly banging and smashing it into things.

After a week of this abuse, it broke open and oozed a pinkish liquid. It was becoming infected, and Louis was getting worried. Before bed, he would hit it with a little hydrogen peroxide, Neosporin cream, and a big fat Band-Aid. Every morning, I would clean the scrape (which was getting worse, not better) and swear that "Today is the day it's going to heal."

As they say: the best laid plans of mice and flesh wounds. The little wound was oozing and glowing angrily. Ten days had passed, yet this thing refused to heal.

"You're getting a front-row seat to what will happen if you catch even a simple cold," Louis said. Less than 24 hours stood between me and the rehearsal. He dabbed peroxide on the freshly opened skin, the white bubbles instantly appearing, along with the expected stabbing needles. "It would take you ten days to get over a three-day cold. That's *if* it doesn't turn into pneumonia."

I knew he was right. My latest white blood cell count had revealed that I was still way below the normal level. Xeloda and Avastin were wreaking havoc on my bone marrow. Regardless of whether I wanted to believe it, the numbers did not lie.

Although I had my own anxieties brewing under the surface about this situation, hearing Louis express his made me dig in my heels. Like a proper donkey, I felt the need to push against his resistance. "I'll be wearing my mask the whole time," I pointed out. "And I won't hug anyone."

He was equally stubborn and was not going to budge. "That won't matter when sitting in a room full of germs being blown out of the ends of instruments," he said matter-of-factly, pressing the Band-Aid onto my skin a little harder than was probably necessary.

Fine. Point taken. This was risky. And for what? So I could avoid boredom and feeling useless? A common cold could turn into something way more serious; COVID was still alive and well, new variations still popping up all the time.

People wanted to believe that just the mere act of being tired of COVID would eradicate it from the world. This virus was going to be with us for a long time, masks or no masks. Was I willing to risk my health for this? Many of the people in the orchestra have to go without masks—playing flutes and trumpets requires mouths. Even those playing instruments that do not involve the face at all were going unmasked. It would mean being in a room for three hours with a lot of people exchanging germs all around me.

It was difficult to make a definitive decision to skip the concert. I was desperate to get back to my normal life. But the risk/reward ratio was tipped too far in the wrong direction.

Turns out, there were a lot of musicians worried on my behalf. The cello section was genuinely stressed about me going to rehearsal. Our concertmaster had texted to tell me she was uncomfortable having me there. I was relieved when the final ruling came down: Pam sent a text at 10 p.m. the night before with her 2-cents.

The text simply said, "I vote no."

Knitting

Survivor's guilt is a complicated, many layered emotional experience for many survivors of cancer. A friend who went through radiation for breast cancer told me she felt guilty for complaining about her side effects to me. "I have no business feeling like this since chemotherapy is so much worse." This is not a contest to see whose treatments are harder. Radiation and chemotherapy are not even on the same playing field. It is about our individual struggle to deal with the physical and mental effects. Although I had a very serious diagnosis, I was doing the same thing. I saw other colon cancer patients with more metastases, more treatments, and more trauma than me. Why am I complaining? I should be thankful for my victories. No matter how guilty I felt, I had to understand my good luck did not come at the expense of anyone else.

Survivor's guilt comes in tiny, subtle waves for me. I look at Suzy sitting across from me in her living room, legs gracefully curled under her on the sofa, her black hair backlit by the sun through the window, giving her an otherworldly appearance, and I wonder, "Why is this beautiful, kind, loving, incredible creature still struggling to beat her cancer?" I may not be saying the obvious end to the sentence—*while I am doing well*—but I feel it the same way I feel certain my dogs will come when I call them, or that my son will text me when he hears a new song he wants to share with me. Why *am* I doing so well? Just like the question about Suzy's setbacks, there is no answer for my victories, either.

I have faced a monumental challenge during cancer: to love and to give of myself freely, even in the face of heartbreak. I had tried so hard to avoid making friends with other cancer patients, and I failed miserably. I allowed myself to become hopelessly attached to Suzy. On its own, that already was too much to bear. Then I met Vicky. And with Vicky, things are different because she is not my age—she is 81. Even without cancer, I know friendships with people that age might not last all that long. Lest I forget, she could still outlive me—the specter of Stage-4C cancer will never again allow me to bask in the full golden light that shines on the innocent certainty of living a long life.

So, when the text comes in from Vicky telling me she is not doing well, her chemotherapy is giving her terrible side effects, and Dr. Jacobs is planning to change around the medications to find a combination that she can tolerate, of course I worry. At our recent appointments, she looked tired, pale, and her hair was thinning. She was no longer getting out of the wheelchair to stand at the nurse's check-in desk like she did just a few weeks ago. I desperately wanted a photo of her before the disease robbed her of her familiar looks. This was how I wanted to remember her—with her long dark hair, round apple cheeks, and bright smile. I would hold on to the photo as the inevitable end closed in a few months later. Right now, she was tired and yet, she was fighting with all the strength she had. I admired her for her grace in the shadow of this horrible disease.

I wondered how often she thought, "This isn't fair!" She never smoked a cigarette in her life, now here she was with lung cancer. She had every right to be angry. Instead, she was cheerful through the fog of the drugs.

"We could be related," she said as we looked through the photos like teenagers reviewing a photo booth printout. We giggled about how much I looked like a younger version of her. I kissed her cheek and pressed my face into her hair. I loved this woman so much that it sometimes hurt. I failed big time—I had allowed myself to become so attached to her I could already feel the cracks forming in my heart.

Usually, when I see Vicky's name pop up on my phone screen, she is texting me to see how I am doing. I always try to pump her for information on her health. But she is remiss to give me details. "Just a little bump in the road," she would respond, but only if I pressed her. I appreciated that she wanted to protect me, but I never wanted to be blindsided. I had also given her an open invitation to let me know if she needed me to run errands or sit with her during infusions. Anything. I would be there for her. She would usually decline, but then say, "I'll let Gary know in case he needs something." I admired her love for her husband and how they put the other person first at every stage of their lives.

But on this day, the text from Vicky made my heart squeeze and my throat tighten. "Sadly, I am hospitalized with a stroke."

I was typing out my response ("Oh no! Would you like company at the hospital? Is Gary ok?") when another text popped up on my screen: "Been having crazy headaches and the back pain has been terrible. For the first time, I feel the cancer is getting ahead of me."

Suzy. She was still waiting to start her next round of chemo. A little over a month ago, she had been hopeful the treatments would begin. Whether it was her insurance making her wait, or scheduling issues with the infusion center, she had been treading water for far too long. The headaches worried me the most, but I would never tell her that.

My heart was being dragged toward the same dark place from two different directions. Both women thought to update me at exactly this moment, and I knew it was just my friendship they needed. Not solutions. Not advice. Just someone to listen to them. I had gotten pretty good at that. I dove into both conversations. I imagined a parallel universe where the three of us were perfectly healthy and texting about meeting this coming

Tuesday morning for coffee and pastries; somewhere there is no cancer, no strokes, no headaches, and there is a perfectly clear blue sky above us.

But in this universe, things are more complicated. I had two friends who needed me in very different, yet eerily similar, ways. Their unspoken needs were coming through loud and clear. It was the same for me during my darkest moments—wanting the company of friends but lacking the energy to have them around. Now I am full of energy, which might be difficult for these two, who are not, to deal with. I was failing them in so many ways, so it astounded me when they continued to include me in their daily briefings.

Every Tuesday, when I receive the Avastin infusions, I can count on seeing Vicky. Our early morning appointments are often one right after the other in Dr. Jacobs' office, so we meet up again in the waiting room before the infusion center opens at 8:30 a.m. Recovering from her stroke, her treatments recommenced. Her hair continued to thin, though she showed no signs of thinning herself. She was as opaque and alive as anyone could be in her situation. Seeing her interact with the nurses, laughing easily as if she were having tea with them, opened my eyes to the difference between people who have a naturally positive energy and those who drag the weight of the world around with them. Vicky was coughing up blood, yet she giggled constantly. She still had more energy and willpower than the cancer. It was important that I did not steal any of her precious energy—she needed to protect her supply. I had more than enough of my own.

One of my colleagues in the orchestra gifted me a box of knitting supplies to occupy my hands and mind while going through radiation treatments last summer. She knew I had been an avid knitter twenty years ago when Andrew was a baby. I had been an expert at knitting baby hats and sweaters for Andrew and for Lori's babies. I even learned to make mittens, socks, and stuffed animals. I had every intention of getting back into the hobby, but never could find the time. She decided it was time for me to knit again. My excitement exploded in a flurry when I saw she had given me full sets of needles in every size of circular, straight, and double-ended—I went on an internet spree of pattern collecting. With this new box of supplies, I could refresh my memory. And within a week, I had started a little assembly line of hats. Vicky was to be my first target.

At night, while Louis and I watched Netflix, I sprawled out on the sofa knitting hats for Vicky. It was fun and easy, and made me feel like I was doing something tangible for her. Knitting resembles meditation. With every stitch there is a count or a pattern—*knit-one, purl-two, knit-one, purl-two, knit-one, purl-two*—to occupy the mind while the body uses muscle memory to complete the task on autopilot. No matter what the hands or mind are doing, the heart is always thinking of the person the knitting is for. Every stitch became *knit-Vicky, purl-Vicky, knit-Vicky, purl-Vicky.* As the hats grew on the needles, so did my courage to keep facing my precarious good health. I never felt sad or worried while knitting. In a few days, the fruit of my labors would sit on her head as a protective layer against the cold outside world.

The weight of Suzy's and Vicky's setbacks sat heavy on my heart. I was doing everything I could not to let their situations dictate my level of happiness. I had so much to be thankful for. Neither Suzy nor Vicky would have been happy to know how much I worried about them. Being able to give them things, though just silly gestures on the surface, made me feel like I was doing something useful.

The Disney Family Cancer Center is a slick, modern building with four floors of integrative cancer treatments. In the ground floor lobby, there is a reflecting pool with a two-story glass-guided water fall that fills the echoey entrance area with the gentle sounds of rain. There is a large seating area, where family often waits while patients finish up their treatments. Behind the row of elevators is the entrance to the radiation department—a labyrinth of hallways and cement structures encasing the arsenal of radiation treatment machines. The third floor is devoted to women's cancers—breast and gynecological cancers. The fourth floor is where I get all my treatments—the PMI Oncology office of Dr. Jacobs on one side of the building, and the infusion center on the other.

Throughout my year of primary treatments, I had not taken advantage of the goodies on the second floor, the home of the Thrivorship Program, where patients and spouses can attend yoga, tai chi, and meditation classes; receive acupuncture and mental health support; visit the hair salon for shaves and wigs; and meet with the nutrition team. During chemo and radiation, I was too tired to drag myself to a class. Now that I was through my primary treatments and on the mend, I was becoming curious about the second floor. Spending just a little time up there, I saw why the patients coming and going from that floor always looked so healthy. I was not the only one who needed these services after the scary treatments were over.

One evening, an email appeared in my inbox. It was from Rémy, the nutritionist who I first met when she was assigned to me during my radiation treatments. She had been integral to my ability to tolerate the IMRT last summer but had also become a trusted advisor and friend. Since my reversal, she had kept up with me, following along with my progress, but also offering warm and important advice for my recovery, both physically and emotionally.

She was writing to tell me about a book launch party taking place on the Second Floor for another young cancer survivor named Traci. Her photo journal, *1 Cancer Patient*, documented her three cancer diagnoses and the life altering treatments that went with them. A few days ahead of the book signing, my copy arrived in the mail. I devoured every page in just under two hours. The photographs were indescribably powerful. She cut straight to the core of what it feels like to be a cancer patient, holding back nothing. She was vulnerable, whether by showing the devastation of the treatments on her body, or the simplicity of standing side by side with her husband, holding hands.

Traci's book was intense; many of the pictures are difficult to look at. The images are universal to all cancer survivors, which she presents in a way that we might use to illustrate what we had gone through ourselves. The photos Louis had taken of me during chemo were of the same basic themes—hair loss, head shaving, moon face, struggling through daily activities, suffering during an infusion—but she turned hers into art.

She included a brief chapter on her sexual dysfunction caused by her treatments. She did not go into deep detail, but the courage needed to call it by its real name in her book showed me just how chicken shit I had been while writing *Round the Twist*—I had not even summoned the minimal amount of courage needed to scratch the surface of what I was going through. I had a laundry list of justifications: the subject was not relevant to the overall story line, the real issues with it did not fully appear until long after my reversal surgery, and did I want my friends, family, and colleagues to know about this very intimate detail of my life? Truth is, this side effect had become a problem during radiation treatments, long before I had my reversal, so that excuse was based on a flat-out lie. Despite knowing other women would benefit from my experience, I was embarrassed and wanted privacy. But not Traci. She threw up her guts onto the page and dared the world to look at the mess.

I was looking forward to meeting her, even if I was feeling a bit star struck. Rémy was the first to recognize me when I stepped out of the elevator into the middle of the launch party. She called me over to a small group of nurses. After quickly catching up on the last nine months of my recovery, she pointed me toward Traci—who was no longer sitting behind the table signing copies of the book but socializing easily with the guests. Sheepishly, I introduced myself, and to my surprise, she pulled me in for a hug. We talked for exactly two minutes before we decided that we absolutely had to spend more time together. She signed the book: "To my new sister," and it ended up being truer than we could have imagined. It felt as if we had known each other our entire lives.

Traci is a part of this wave of young women under 50 with cancer. First diagnosed at 39 with breast cancer, she overcame that only to be hit two more times with metastatic cancer—first to her cervical spine, next to her brain. Traci is doing a lot more than just surviving these multiple onslaughts. She is thriving. She shows no sign of giving up or giving in; she is not resigned to her fate; and she absolutely does not live in fear. Cancer and all the treatments have ravaged her petite body. Yet, there she sat across the table from me a week later, strong, and laughing as if she had no cares in the world.

We discovered we had so much in common. It really was like we were sisters separated at birth. Only months apart in age, we are the same height, are both vegans, and practice yoga. We both wore black shirts, dark jeans, and sneakers (me in my favorite maroon Vans, she in her navy-blue Chucks). We spent a bit of time comparing all our tattoos and laughing about how we were both wearing grey socks.

Munching happily on a vegan sandwich was someone who had every right to be angry, bitter, and discouraged. And yet, she was vibrant, positive, and joyful. From where I sat, it was clear she did not base her happiness on the success of other people's private battles with cancer. And not because she is heartless or unfeeling, but because she is one person. She is, as I was coming to see for myself, one unique person whose survival is not dependent on anyone but herself. She could be fully engaged with another cancer survivor, hear their story, and celebrate.

And I believe, if she needed to, she could also mourn with heartbreaking empathy.

Our conversation was easy and light. We spent nearly five hours together, laughing like old friends, and comparing our cancer journeys. It was easy to talk about all the very private things that happened to us during our treatments. She encouraged me to get a laser treatment from my gynecologist, because she had tried it and it changed her world. More than anything, we needed someone to talk to about how our lives had changed because of cancer—how it changed some relationships for the better, ended some completely, and left others in a fractured state worse than broken.

We talked for so long our server's shift ended. We moved to the patio furniture around the fire table and ordered coffee and tea. We had to leave before rush hour traffic, otherwise the conversation would have never ended. We hugged goodbye in the parking lot, then hugged again next to my car. We waved at each other as she walked to her car, and I drove by in mine.

What I had just witnessed in Traci was an island before me. Solid. Vibrant. *Alive.* I am all those things, too. Vicky does not need me to feel sorry for her. Suzy does not need me to feel guilty. What they needed from me was exactly what I got from Traci—a friend who was so strong that I could be an island, too. On my island, Vicky and Suzy could lie on the beach, under my solitary palm tree, and take in some life-giving sunshine. Alone-Together is not about despairing in individual bubbles, it is about circling the same bright nucleus called Hope.

In the weeks that followed, we made more lunch dates, more plans, shared texts and emails, laughed at each other's jokes on Facebook, and promoted each other's books. She continued to put out video compilations filmed during her treatments—one that hit me the hardest was a black and white montage of shaving her head after her third diagnosis. It is dark, stormy, hopeful, and heartbreaking—the visual effects giving one the impression that they are peering into an actual memory playing inside her mind. Once her head is shaved, her face, which had been brave and tough up to this point, flashed a childlike uncertainty. It reminded me of Andrew's first day of kindergarten, except Traci didn't have to wonder—she knew for sure cancer was the monster waiting behind the door.

The image flashed on the screen, and I sucked in an involuntary breath, gasping suddenly in the silent room. Louis sat forward, grabbed my arm, and immediately asked if I was ok. "Does something hurt?" He was still on high alert—on the lookout for bouts of pain that might signal new cancer. We were both on edge after what we had gone through.

I showed him the video of Traci shaving her head, and when I heard him sniffle, I knew he had recognized the same expression that had affected me so deeply.

"I know you," the words that I had written so long ago to describe cancer patients gazing at each other.

In just a year, I had added three new friends to my little tribe, like colorful yarn knitted together to form a protective blanket. Were it not for cancer, we would have never met. My little coven was now four women strong. This fight did not need black magic. We just needed each other.

The Big Owie

The gynecological side-effects of radiation and chemotherapy can be a highly embarrassing subject for women cancer survivors to talk about. Many women have hysterectomies or loose one or both ovaries during their cancer treatments, causing another set of issues. Because I had no idea what to expect when I began treatments, I took my side effects for granted. I also assumed that every woman had them and that there was nothing to be done about them. Talking about these side-effects seemed like an indulgence—I had heard none of my women survivor friends ever mention anything like these side-effects, which led me to believe that I was just being weak. I believed I needed to chin up and soldier through in silence.

But, in this year since radiation ended, I learned I am not alone. Women just do not talk about it—either with each other or with their doctors. Many just accept what happened to them and assume there is nothing to be done for it. Men who have radiation for pelvic cancers are warned about erectile dysfunction—though they may not talk openly about it either. But, like many women under 50, I had no clue this thing could happen to me after cancer treatments.

Colon cancer has historically affected older adults in their 70s, which, although it may leave them with the same physical effects I experienced, it may not affect them the same way emotionally. With the recent wave of young women being diagnosed with colon cancer before menopause, discussing the short-term and lasting effects with our doctors, support system, and other women survivors is crucial.

I wish I had been better prepared. Of course, the bilateral salpingo oophorectomy (removal of both fallopian tubes and ovaries) ensured I would go through menopause. Beyond that, no one seemed all that certain what other long-term effects chemo or radiation might have on me. Unfortunately, we would not know the full extent of the damage until long after I finished radiation and fully recovered from my colostomy reversal surgery—six months would pass before I could resume normal physical activities like yoga and running. That included sex. Everyone—me, my oncology team, the nurses, my gynecologist, my husband—were waiting with bated breath to see what had actually happened to me.

Doctors inform both male and female patients that chemotherapy might cause infertility. I had been duly warned my drugs would have this side effect. Before treatments begin, men may choose to freeze their sperm and women may have eggs harvested. In our case, Louis and I were long finished having children—all three of our boys were in their 20s—so I welcomed infertility and menopause with open arms.

At the time of my colectomy, the surgeon removed my left ovary—it had blown up to 13cm (the size of a grapefruit) because of the colon cancer which had metastasized onto it. The next morning, I had the expected vaginal bleeding. This would be the last time I had anything that even remotely resembled a period ever again. During my hospital stay, I had severe hot flashes each day, and at night I soaked my hospital bed with sweat, my hair damp and clinging to my neck. And then it was over—the fabled change of life took less than 72 hours to complete. Chemotherapy began four weeks later, and the remaining ovary was officially closed for business.

Three months later, when chemotherapy ended, my body gave no sign of returning menses. I spent a lot of time joking that this was the only side effect of chemo I had looked forward to. I still had a hormone IUD, which was undoubtedly helping a bit with the lingering symptoms of this medical menopause. So that it did not melt into my uterus, the IUD had to be removed before radiation.

Knowing that the cancer the surgeon left behind was sitting between my vagina and rectum, Louis and I decided we would refrain from any sexual activity. We imagined the cancer exploding and bathing my pelvis in free-floating metastatic cells. I had also read that with some chemotherapy drugs, there is a slight possibility of exposing your partner to the toxicity of the drugs, and I was unwilling to put Louis in that position. Besides, chemotherapy was tough enough—who has the energy for anything else? Not me. Louis was exhausted from worrying and taking care of me; we had more important things on our minds. After my diagnosis, and during all of my treatments, affection and closeness became a major priority. In fact, I think we became even closer as a couple during this period.

Just before I began the Intensity Modulated Radiation Therapy (IMRT), all the doctors and nurses reiterated that infertility would be unavoidable. They also informed me I would experience some level of sexual dysfunction thanks to the X-rays bombarding my pelvis. Although IMRT might spare delicate tissues and mostly target the cancer, it would bathe my entire abdomen from the base of my sternum to my pelvic bone in radiation. The radiation treatment would cook my insides, broiling and boiling everything in its path, reproductive organs included. Most of the digestive organs would heal and return to normal function within a few months. There remained a big question mark next to the vagina because the IMRT would hit it directly in an attempt to zap the remaining cancer cells that had been left behind after chemo. Even before IMRT did its damage, the primary cancer had already threatened my vagina and rectum, the disease might have left the two organs severely and irreparably damaged anyway. In the end, the surgeon might have to remove both when this was over, leaving me with a permanent colostomy, no rectum, and no vagina.

Would the scar tissue forming in my pelvis from the IMRT strangle and crush the delicate vagina? Would it collapse in on itself and become utterly useless? If I were of the average age of female colon cancer patients (72), this might not be at the top of my worry list. But at 48, I was not ready to close up shop.

"You should attempt to have intercourse as often as possible during treatment," Dr. Menzel, my radiation oncologist, advised Louis and me in the days before treatment began. "We want to prevent a stricture, and if you can dilate the muscles, you may prevent this." This was the first time I had ever heard of such a thing. I would have to take this seriously.

"Prescription sex? He's the best doctor ever!" Louis joked in the car on the way home. We dove in enthusiastically, like a couple of newlyweds, fully intending to follow Dr. Menzel's advice. Nurse Cindy questioned me about our progress at my first two weekly check-ins, her questions centered on my pain level—which at that early stage was nothing.

Louis and I were taking our homework seriously, and it was a lot of fun. But as the days marched on, and the treatments began taking their toll on my body, I was losing my enthusiasm for expending the extra energy. The damage was already beginning to appear, and it was becoming more and more painful. Around the 3-week mark, we had to stop. The pain was unbearable, and I cried at the mere thought of trying.

We made the tough decision to stop. We knew that more damage was going to occur before IMRT ended. How bad would it be when the treatment was over? By giving up now, we were taking a huge gamble. It would be months after reversal surgery before we could begin trying again. Only then would we know if we had given up too soon. I was stressed and worried, not knowing what awaited me at the end of our abstinence. It is one thing to be patient about getting back to yoga or hiking—hamstrings and abs are large muscles that can handle quite a bit of discomfort. The vagina is sensitive and delicate, and not a body part used to pain. Terrible things were most likely waiting for me in the future.

Cindy was my greatest source of comfort and support. I had a check-up with Dr. Menzel one month after my ostomy reversal surgery. It did not discourage Cindy. She was confident that a dilator would help—I might even be one of the lucky women who avoids any additional treatments. I desperately wanted her to be right.

One month into the process, I was already frustrated and worried. Was anything actually happening? Was anything getting fixed or was I just spinning my wheels? A long phone call with Cindy, in which we talked about the slow progress I was making, offered me some reassurance. She recommended I see my gynecologist to get a proper look at what was going on. She reminded me not to panic, and to be patient with my body—it had been through a lot, and stressing myself out would solve nothing.

I worried that the damage may not be reversible. While I messed around with these dilators, was the damage becoming permanent? Was this one of those things where the longer it persisted, the harder it was to fix? I was angry cancer had stripped us of one of the most important aspects of a healthy marriage. Was there any point in trying to fix this? It was so painful and slow, with no guarantees waiting at the end. Maybe I should give up and just accept my fate.

Five months later, in April, I met with Cindy and Dr. Menzel for my 9-month post-radiation check-up. Besides confirming what I already knew for myself—that I had mostly healed physically from the IMRT—they were both more interested in the long-term effects of the treatment on a younger patient.

"Most of what we know about the lasting effects of IMRT therapies has to do with older patients in their 70s and 80s. These are people for whom sexual dysfunction may not be a top concern. Treating people in their 40s, or younger, is new territory for most of us," Dr. Menzel was explaining why the heightened curiosity regarding my lasting effects was so important for his own notes. I wondered if my vagina was about to appear in some medical journal.

During this appointment, he also informed me that IMRT is not normally administered to as large an area as I was given, so he was especially interested in my physical recovery. Was I still having abdominal pain? How long did it take for the diarrhea to subside after my colostomy reversal? How long before I was eating a normal diet? Was 8 weeks post-op long enough to recover before resuming my normal exercise routines? And, always an important question, what was my daily bowel routine like now? I imagined Dr. Menzel sitting at his computer after our appointment recounting the information I eagerly gave in answer to all those questions. I wasn't shy with either Dr. Menzel or Cindy, because their interest was not just clinical, it was also compassionate. At one point in our discussion, he was apologetic about his unrelenting inquiries, but I simply said, "I wrote a book with all the gory details. I'm not shy about answering any of your questions!"

My answers would help shape the way they approached the long-term treatment of future young women cancer patients, which was why I took this interview seriously.

The doctors told me to be persistent and patient with my recovery. Still, I felt a lot of stress and guilt for Louis. What person signs up for a sexless marriage? No matter how many times he said, "You're alive, and that's all I care about," I just felt like a flat-out failure.

None of this was fair. It hurt so badly; I wanted to avoid the whole thing. Just the thought of intercourse would send a jolt of horror through my body. I was resentful that cancer had taken this pleasure from my husband and angry that I had to work this hard to fix it. I felt defeated. *I wouldn't care if I never had sex again,* I admitted to myself one day. What an awful thing to think. Now, on top of everything else, I felt ungrateful. I was surviving Stage-4C cancer against the odds, only to live a sexless life? My anger was aimed at a side effect of survival, adding more fuel to my fire of guilt. I should be thankful to be alive. Instead, I was complaining.

The physical aspect of the issue was the straightforward part. The emotional part was the most difficult to deal with. When I finally started seeing a therapist, we discussed this issue at great length. She had also survived colon cancer, but unlike me, there were no treatments for the damage done to her body. It was the first time I spoke with someone who truly understood. She was not just an empathetic listener, trying to soothe me. She was living it.

"What are you feeling right now?" she asked me. Sitting across from her, staring out the window at the Zen garden in the courtyard of the DFCC, I tried desperately not to cry. She had suggested I imagine I would have sex that night, and what sort of reaction was I having to that idea?

"I'm scared and angry. I also feel guilty and like I'm a failure." I took a breath and blinked back the tears. "I know how much it's going to hurt and I feel sick just thinking about it. That's how scared I feel right now." I brought my hand to my solar plexus. "It hurts right here." I don't know who it was harder to admit these things to: my husband, my therapist, or myself.

Almost exactly one year after chemotherapy ended, my gynecologist Dr. Silberstein was doing yet another a pelvic exam, careful not to cause too much pain and discomfort. "You don't have any ovaries, so don't forget that on top of all the treatments, you've also gone through menopause," she explained when I could sit in a more dignified position. "Your body doesn't make the same hormones that it used to, and that means that the pain you're feeling is mostly from friction, not from the muscles themselves."

The tissues and muscles around the vagina were just fine. It was my lack of hormones that was causing the problem. Fortunately, there are simple treatments for this. First, she prescribed low dose hormones, since I was too young to be in menopause. She suggested a laser treatment that would help build up more elastic tissue in the vagina. Our insurance would not cover it, but the high cost seemed like a small price to pay. After discussing all this with Traci, my trusted advisor in female cancer matters, I was back in Dr. Silberstein's office for the first of three laser treatments.

The process itself was not painful—it was mildly irritating. By the time she declared, "We're halfway through," it surprised me how quickly it was going. For a few hours following the treatment, I was more comfortable standing up than sitting down. But by the time I went to bed, there was barely any hint that anything had happened at all.

It was time to test out the results, and we were up to the task. But by this point, I was jumpy and nervous. Most of what I was feeling had more to do with emotional baggage than actual physical issues. So, with a lot of patience and understanding, we made our first careful attempts. The effects of the three treatments were noticeable. For the first time in nearly a year, I had hope. It was a tremendous relief for my head and heart. And fixing the physical pain was key to the emotional side of the healing process.

By telling my story, I want to give other women hope. There are ways to fix what has happened to your body, but it takes patience and compassion. But I also hope that oncologists and other medical professionals learn more about this and are able to present more options to younger women. It is important they tell women about these side effects early on, giving them time to research the options so they can line up their follow-up treatments as soon as possible.

When I was brave enough to break my silence, I discovered I was never really alone. Women need to hear my story. Although it will be weird to know everyone now knows many intimate details of my life, I had to remember when I was going through this, I had no one to turn to. So, to the other women reading this who are going through the same thing, know that you are not alone. You are not unique. And I know exactly how you are feeling.

Author's Note: The treatment that I had is sometimes called "Mona Lisa Touch" and is used to rejuvenate post-menopausal vaginal tissue. The laser breaks down tissue, potentially resulting in thicker and more flexible regrowth. Most insurance policies do not cover the cost of this treatment, making it prohibitive for many women. It worked for me, so I consider it a wise investment. If you have painful intercourse because of menopause, chemotherapy, radiation, hysterectomy, or oophorectomy, talk to your gynecologist about this option.

Bell Day

For the first time in several months, Louis' morning schedule was clear; today we would hike as a team. The last time we were out there together, Louis had taken me to one of his favorite trails. With him in charge of the hike, I was a passenger with no responsibility other than to enjoy the scenery.

But today was different. It was March 18, 2023. Exactly one year ago, I rang the bell, signifying the end of my chemotherapy treatments. Even after all this time, I was hard to believe I had completed chemotherapy. *Me. I did that.* Because of these lingering thoughts, I had trouble sleeping, waking often during the night, my legs restless, and my mind racing. The sound of the phantom 5-FU pump played in the dark, punctuating the memories cycling through my mind.

I was out of bed long before Louis. The first hint of sunrise is my signal to get the day started. I always wake up with the dawn, which usually works out great. But Daylight Savings kicked in last weekend; my internal clock had not adjusted to be in sync with the numbers on my watch. The lost hour brought with it unnecessary exhaustion, as I still needed to take my Xeloda pill on a tight 12-hour schedule. I was not yet going to bed early enough to even out the morning wake-up. This week, I started each day just a little more tired than the one before.

No matter. I would finish this cycle of Xeloda this weekend, then I could sleep a few extra minutes. It would make a huge difference once my body could wake itself in a more natural way. Of course, assuming the dogs left me alone. Even if Louis were to get up to let them out, they would still come back to jump on the bed and lick my ears sticking out from the blankets. I'm always delighted by this, no matter how tired I am. "Hooray hooray! A brand-new day!" The dogs romp and howl when I cheer this every morning.

I began the morning as usual: setting the teakettle to boil while I unloaded the dishwasher and fed the dogs. I watered my beloved Venus flytraps—during chemo, I collected several of the carnivorous plants, and named them all *Audrey* (after the musical, of course). My obsession threatened to turn me into the *Crazy Venus Flytrap Lady*. After saying good morning to each and every one of my *Audreys* on the window shelf, I took my place on the sofa to sip my tea, play Wordle, and watch CNN. The news about the ongoing invasion of Ukraine was just too sad, so I turned to TLC, where there is always some disgusting medical show like *Dr. Pimple Popper* or outrageous reality series like *90 Day Fiancé* to distract me from the horrors of the real world. I nibbled a handful of saltine crackers before swallowing my morning dose of Xeloda, and as always, I wished it luck before I washed it down.

It was time to face this strange anniversary. I started by looking through my phone at photos Louis had taken of me during chemo, but especially at the photos of the last days. The final infusion had been the worst of all six—bringing the most intense fatigue, the worst of the mouth sores, and peeling skin. These were just the things I could remember—my memory was so hazy from chemo. If I had not written down all my side effects as they were happening, I would have forgotten them all. I stopped scrolling when I saw the picture of bald me flashing a thumbs-up—the IV had just been disconnected from my portacath, and I was waiting to ring the bell.

My nurses, Abby and Terry, were not there that particular Friday. Normally, they were the ones who disconnected me from the pump. If they had been there, they would have made a bigger fuss about my final infusion. But they had the day off, so I had another nurse who was unaware this was my last day. She simply removed the IV, flushed the port, and then wished me a good weekend.

"Today is her last day," Louis said, a little anxious that this momentous day might go uncelebrated. She apologized for not knowing. A few minutes later, she returned with the bell and a certificate, followed by several of the other infusion nurses who *did* know what day this was.

"Congratulations!!!" they all cheered. As I rang my bell, other patients clapped from their cubicles. I was disappointed Terry and Abby were not there to share this moment with me. But I was thankful Louis had stepped in to fix this when I was too exhausted and foggy to realize what was happening.

"So, what are you up to today?" Louis asked, his voice pulling me back into the present as he settled on the sofa next to me, his coffee mug in hand.

"I'm going for a hike," I said. "I need to be on the mountain. This is 'Bell Day'."

"Oh right! I assume you plan to go alone?" He understood I needed solitude once in a while, and often when I went hiking as opposed to practicing yoga, it signaled that I needed private time.

"Actually," I said, getting a little teary. "I think you need to be with me for this."

He patted my leg tenderly. "I know it's a strange day."

About a week before this, Louis decided he would make a video for me to post on my website, YouTube, and social media to promote the book. He bought some new software and, when he should have been working on his actual job, he was creating this book-trailer video for me. He pulled together many photos and videos of me during chemotherapy, radiation treatments, and going through the various stages of recovery from surgeries. The final touch was a very sweet piece of music he wrote, which plays over the whole thing. When he showed the first demo version to me, I burst out crying.

"I know, it's really hard to see yourself like that," he whispered, holding me while I sobbed out loud into his chest.

"I still can't believe any of this!" Was I crying because the images were intense or because this thing had happened at all?

We decided we needed more uplifting videos of me for the final version of the trailer. Positive images of me recovered interspersed with the cancer treatments, since the book was about the power of positivity and not about suffering. While we were hiking today, we would get more videos.

What I really wanted was a photo of me celebrating the anniversary. I put together a collage of photos from the last day of chemo—the certificate, the thumbs-up photo, and a picture of me with the pump—to post to my social media. No less than five minutes passed before people were commenting and liking the post. Probably like me, those people who truly know me also had a hard time believing that an entire year had already passed. It felt as if chemo had only ended last week, and in other ways, as if it had happened 20 years ago.

On today's hike, I would be in charge of choosing the route, and I wanted to go on one of my favorite trails. Even before COVID, I was probably one of very few people who used this very remote trail with any frequency. While the park was closed for several months during the lockdown, the trail became overgrown. Since then, of course some maintenance had happened, which meant the trail was mostly open. Although, there was still a stretch of about 50 yards that required some bravery to keep moving forward—the trail was nearly invisible under the tall green grasses and overgrown weeds.

I led the way, my sure feet breaking through the grasses of the familiar path. I carefully picked my way down a sheer rock and then crossed a rushing stream. The trail winds its way down the mountain, eventually connecting with the Miranda Trail. We would have to pass through the destruction scar on my beloved *Miranda*. It filled me with fresh indignation and outrage, just as strong as the day the dogs and I discovered it. After two years, the land still struggled to heal.

From this vantage point, the burn area was clearly visible in the park below. It was full of wildflowers and grasses. It was hard to believe there had been a fire at all. That land was healing and thriving. But not *Miranda*. The chaparral and grasses were still struggling to get a foothold; the manzanita were not throwing up shoots; the landscape looked sickly and beige. Mother Nature does not give up, though. Things would grow back. I was sure of it. It would simply take longer than in the burn. *Miranda* would always carry scars, even if the plant-life grew to cover them.

As we passed through, I basked in the kinship I felt with the land that a human cancer had ravaged. My body was put back together, but the damaged edges had not quite blended with the healthy skin around them. I had a lot of energy, but my reserves were always running low. The weeds were not as lush as in the rest of the park, but at least they covered the bare dirt. Nature was trying her best to erase all signs of the attack. The Earth wanted to forget. *Miranda* wanted to forget. I wanted to forget.

With each footstep through the scar, I could feel she recognized me as a fellow survivor. We were both transformed; no longer the same trusting spirits we were before. We had been wounded, and we would not soon forget. Just off the trail, I climbed a pile of boulders. Standing tall, I looked out at the valley stretched out below. Hands on my hips, I stared out, contemplating the hills and trails and trees. I turned back to face Louis, and he snapped a few pictures of me raising my arms above my head.

I am alive.

Part 3

"Hooray hooray, a brand-new day!"
–Dusty & Luna

Challenge Accepted

My prodigal run as an advancing high school oboist had reached its first major milestone: college auditions. Compared to the other 12th grade applicants, I was five years behind in my training. I needed to make up a lot of ground if I wanted a shot at a reputable college. My band director had set me up with private lessons with her husband, a professional oboist. We all believed that our combined efforts could get me into any college I wanted—I just had to practice, stay focused, and not fall on my face during the auditions.

When I attended Ithaca College in the early 1990s, the music department was a tiny, tight-knit community of students. I worked my ass off all four years. Every night was a late night for me, practicing until the janitor locked up at 1 a.m. My friend Jeremy and I would choose adjacent practice rooms to good-naturedly outplay the other through the thin walls. The oboe studio was exceptionally close, more like a family than anything else. We would spend hours together in the Reed Room—the workshop where we made our reeds. But more importantly, it was the place where we laughed, drank smuggled box wine, and built lifelong bonds.

By the time we graduated, I was engaged to a fellow oboist named Matt. He had a job offer that would require us to move back to his hometown of Williamstown, Massachusetts, the picturesque New England town nestled in the Berkshire mountains. Because of its central location, there were also plenty of musical opportunities for me in nearby New York and

Vermont. I was busy almost every weekend with some sort of concert. We spent nine years in Williamstown. Although we had started out full of hope, our marriage was already on the rocks long before Andrew was born. The more years we spent together, the worse it was getting. In what would be our last act of marital cooperation, we made a radical change: *Viva Las Vegas!*

Amidst a flurry of tears, we pulled up stakes and headed west. As a teacher, Matt had no problem finding a job right away. But I arrived with no prospects—just a collection of instruments and the hope that I might catch a break. With no contacts, I did the only sensible thing: I called the oboe professor at the University of Nevada, Las Vegas, and asked for advice. He invited me to meet at his office, where we spent the afternoon playing duets and getting to know each other. "The woman who plays oboe in *The Phantom of the Opera* went to Ithaca College, too," he informed me. "I wonder if you know Yvonne?"

Did I know her? She had been one of my closest friends. But these were the days before social media, so we had lost contact shortly after graduation ten years earlier. He gave me her phone number, and later that day when her familiar voice answered, I exclaimed, "Hey bitch, guess who's in town?"

The shrieks that came back through the phone nearly deafened me. Everything was going to be alright. Yvonne was here.

Deciding to split up after twelve years of marriage was fraught with wild emotions and explosive arguments. The animosity and resentment had been growing for over a decade. After a year of sleeping in separate bedrooms, the outward manifestation of those things, Matt and I came to the painful acceptance of the only solution: divorce.

During the divorce process, I found life as a single mother to a 7-year-old to be even harder than I had expected. I cannot recall a single restful night's sleep in the year after the divorce. I would have to make enough money to support Andrew by myself. Since my only actual skills were in music, I had to be the best musician possible, hoping it would be enough.

For several months, I had been doing recording work for Louis, a tv composer who lived in Los Angeles. I was good at it, and he seemed pleased with my playing. He was hiring me week after week, and I was getting a taste of what it felt like to use my skills. He gave me the confidence that I might make a living doing this very fun and interesting thing.

An oboist friend in Los Angeles decided it was time for me and Louis to meet in person, so he invited us both to a party he was throwing. Finally, I would meet the man I had been working for (all our interactions up to this point were over email and the phone). I made the four-hour drive across the desert. Louis spotted me in the crowd and made straight for me. He wrapped me up in his arms and I swear it felt as if we already knew each other. We went off into a quiet corner of the patio and talked by the space heater. Never missing a beat, the conversation would continue uninterrupted for the rest of our lives.

"Want to get out of here?" He tempted, his fingertips lightly touching my wrist.

"Let's go!" I jumped up, and we were in his car on our way to drinks. The dive bar left no impression on me, but I remember I had wanted to take his hand as we walked back out to his car two hours later.

I was in town for three days, and we spent all three days together. I hardly remember anything else except Louis' deep voice close to my ear in a jazz club, my first mojito, and the way he would touch my fingers when he spoke to me.

We dated for several months before he suggested I move to Los Angeles to be with him. Andrew and I packed up our belongings and our cat and left Las Vegas. It was exciting to be in the new city. Andrew was adjusting to his new school, and

Louis was helping me get some work. Things were coming together again.

"Did you hear that Bennett died on stage last night?" Bob, the second oboist, said dolefully, as I took my seat beside him on stage. William Bennett was the well-respected, much loved oboist with the San Francisco Symphony. "Rumor is that he had a stroke on stage while performing the Strauss Concerto," Bob continued as we assembled our oboes.

This was terrible news, but all of us oboists live with the specter of serious injury looming over us. The strength it takes to blow so hard through the tiny oboe reed causes all kinds of injuries. It is only a matter of time before these stories come down the pipeline. What Bob did not know was I was hiding my own oboe-related injury from everyone on the stage.

A year and a half before this conversation, I felt something give way in my abdomen during a concert. Suddenly, I could not play as loud as I was used to. There was no strength or power behind my playing—my abdomen felt useless. But, as the saying goes, the show must go on.

When the concert ended, Bob noticed a bulge in my belly pushing through my shirt when I stood up for my solo bow. "Did you always have that?" he asked when the stage lights had gone down, and we could talk under the noise of the other musicians as they packed up.

I shrugged. "I have no idea. What do you think it is?" I poked at the new little bump. "Weird, right?"

Bob made a face that did not make me feel any better. No matter. I had more performances that autumn and no time for doctors' appointments and tests. Besides, it didn't hurt. It must not be that serious, whatever it was.

I played with that hernia for eighteen months. I was still so new to the Los Angeles music scene, there was never a good time to take a break for a surgery. My biggest fear was the hernia reopening when I played my oboe again, the very thing that caused the initial injury. I faced a choice: risk damaging the repair or give up the oboe forever.

"Count yourself lucky that this is all that happened to you," my former oboe teacher wrote in an email a few months ahead of my repair surgery. "You're an excellent musician, you don't need to be an oboist. Just go out and be a musician."

I thought long and hard about his advice. "Just be a musician," seemed doable.

Deflated and sad at this unexpected detour, I was at a loss for what to do next. "You're always talking about how you wished you played the cello. Why don't you do that?" Louis had made an utterly ridiculous suggestion. No one, and I mean *no one*, ever makes a switch from a woodwind instrument like the oboe to a string instrument like a cello, two completely unrelated instruments—and at my age! Despite my misgivings, we threw down a few hundred dollars to buy a cheap student cello, anticipating I would just learn a few basics from the Suzuki books and happily amuse myself with the instrument alone at home.

My colleague, Pam, offered to give me some lessons to get started, but the moment she heard me play, she had other ideas. "You know, if you devoted all your time to this, you could actually become a cellist."

"For real?" I asked her. "Because it's probably too late for me to do anything but have fun with it."

She never jokes about these kinds of things. "Yes, for real. You could play in the orchestra next year if you set your mind to it."

Challenge accepted.

Louis and I went cello hunting. Like for a real cello this time. Pam and I met every Sunday morning for lessons, and I devoted three hours every single day to practicing. I was hopelessly devoted to this instrument. The first time I saw a real orchestra in concert as a child, I could not stop staring at the cellos in the front of the stage. I wanted to play the cello, but our school did not have a string program. Besides, my parents had spent all that money on my piano, a cello would have been another expense for them. The obsession with the cello persisted my entire life. I was in love with something I thought I could never have—I was Brahms, and the cello was my Clara.

This unexpected injury was forcing me to take stock of my life and career. My new cello, a professional grade beauty, was my constant companion. For the first time in my musical life, I felt I was finally doing something that I truly loved. I proved to myself that I could do amazing things when I set aside fear and uncertainty.

Sunbeams

It felt like every week since October was going by faster and faster, accelerating until suddenly it was springtime. Each round of this chemotherapy was three weeks long, giving the impression of shortened months. My life carved up into this three-week routine where the first two weeks on the drug moved at a frustratingly slow speed, while the third week off the drugs barreled past me in streaking colors. I tried very hard not to schedule things on my week off. I wanted to enjoy reading on the patio, doing yoga and hiking as long as I wanted without a deadline.

"I thought you were already working again," Dr. Jacobs had responded when I asked if it was safe for me to return to rehearsals with the orchestra.

I shook my head. "Oh no. And not because I didn't want to. It's just that our orchestra only gives four concerts each season, and there weren't any concerts going on yet."

This was a wildly distorted version of the truth. The fact was, I had backed out of the fall season of concerts, including the holiday concert, out of fear. But I would not tell him that. I had given up all these recent opportunities because I questioned whether I was truly ready to be back among the living. I had planned on performing in the spring cycle of concerts, and yet I had backed out of the March concert. Now, I promised myself I would play the last concert of the season, the day before my birthday in May, no more excuses. The excitement of performing was building, very different from the trepidation I had been feeling months before.

"Feel free to get back to work," Dr. Jacobs approved. "Maybe continue to wear your mask, though."

"She will," Louis piped up from his chair in the corner. "I don't let her go anywhere without it." I indulged myself in an affectionate eye roll for these two men.

What Dr. Jacobs did not know was how many orchestra members were contacting me to encourage me to get back to playing, and also to remind me to wear my mask all the time. Many people even suggested they would wear masks, knowing they would sit near me in the string section. All that intense positivity of my friends that I enjoyed during chemo and radiation was still coming at me, loud and clear. I felt precious. I felt loved. Everyone I had come in contact with for the last eighteen months was still invested in my well-being. Louis and Dr. Jacobs were always running first and second in that competition.

My first rehearsal in a year and a half was just around the corner. I was practicing my cello as much as I could. The lingering joint pain from chemo was showing up as a nagging ache in my left shoulder—the arm must stay elevated every moment of playing the cello. My bow arm (right arm) has the relief of different movements and angles to offset any discomfort I might sometimes feel. My left shoulder was aching so much now that it even hurt to lie on it in bed. Exactly one week before the first rehearsal, while practicing my cello, I took my left hand down from the fingerboard and lowered my arm. My shoulder gave a loud *crack!* which at first felt good. More worrisome was that my wrist was screaming in agony. My first instinct was to panic—it wasn't so long ago that an unexpected hernia had ended my oboe career. As a musician, even a minor injury could limit my ability to play, making performing an ordeal.

"Well, that's new," I said to the dogs, who had been napping next to my chair while I practiced. The sound of the crack had awakened them both. Dusty had gotten up and stood next to me when he heard me speak, so I showed him my hand. Maybe he knew what was wrong? He didn't, but he licked my fingertips anyway, which made me feel a little better. Luna had no opinion on the matter; she yawned, stretched, shot me an annoyed look for waking her up, and quietly slipped from the room. I patted Dusty's head. "Thanks for caring, Pooper," I smiled down at him. His dark brown eyes holding my gaze, awaiting further instructions. Maybe a thousand of his little licks could cure my sore wrist. In the meantime, I would try some Advil and hope for the best.

Louis was no stranger to my moaning about every minor ache and pain. Unlike me, he has a great bedside manner and is full of empathy and sympathy at the first sign of my distress. We ate dinner and watched Netflix all evening, while I massaged my wrist and worried out loud about this being an issue at the rehearsal next week. Maybe I should back out of this concert, too. Just keep resting. Maybe this is the sign that I am not ready to get back to work.

But it *was* time to get back to real life. No more sitting around, hiding from the world, and hiding from my life. I was afraid of having to hug people, and yet I was dying to feel that affection again. "Life is too short not to hug," I had made a habit of saying to friends when they asked if it was safe to do so. They saw me as breakable, delicate, and vulnerable, which was how I began seeing myself as well. But saying the words, "Life is too short not to hug," inspired me to launch into their arms and genuinely appreciate their presence.

The wrist pain subsided within 24 hours, although the shoulder persisted with no change. Because of all those little pains, I was taking a break from practicing yoga. I was throwing myself into editing the manuscript of a fellow author and working on this book. I had created plenty of busy work to distract myself. As I wrote about my current life, I could take a step back. The space allowed me to sit with the complicated emotions involved in returning to my life. Through this process, I came to discover I was the one creating resistance in my mind. There was no physical reason to sit out anymore. If I waited for myself to take the first step, I would never do it. I had run out of excuses. It was time to rejoin the world.

Flush with the excitement of getting back to practicing for the first rehearsal, I visualized unloading my blue cello case from the Subaru, rolling into the rehearsal, and taking my seat. I would, for the first time in over a year, feel the pure power of a live orchestra jammed into a room barely big enough to hold it. The oboe gives the "A" and everyone joins in to tune, each instrument adding its own unique voice to the mix—hints of the music we are about to play breaking through the cacophony like sunbeams through storm clouds. The expectant energy is wildly palpable. The excitement of this universal orchestral ritual has always excited me. I needed to tap into that energy to keep myself focused on getting back to performing.

A text notification on my phone snapped me back to reality. Suzy. I hesitated, staring at the notification which displayed just a snippet of the first line: "Looks like my surgery is canceled…" I knew in my gut why the surgery was canceled, but the feeling of dread prevented me from opening the text—doing so would make this real.

After a few weeks of testing and more scans of the new mass, the surgeon decided to officially cancel her sigmoidectomy. The new tumor would have to be treated before he could go digging around inside of her. How can this be happening? How can this cancer just continue to grow despite all of the treatments she had gone through the past year and a half? Her news made me realize that although I was in seemingly in good health after several clear scans, I could easily find myself in her position—

something new suddenly appearing out of nowhere. Her intuition had told her something was wrong. And as we have all learned, always listen to that little voice that says *are you sure?*

To lighten our spirits, we met for lunch to catch up and enjoy some unseasonably warm weather. It felt great to sit in the restaurant's patio dining area and feel the warm sun on our necks. Everything seems less scary when sitting in the sunshine. We took advantage of this opportunity to soak in some of these life-giving rays—even if we were supposed to be avoiding the sun while on Xeloda. We did not keep our laughter to ourselves. The opinions of the other patrons of the restaurant mattered little to us. Most people will never fully appreciate just how wonderful it is to be alive on a random Thursday.

Eventually, the laughter tapered off, and Suzy's mood turned dark. Her eyes welled with tears. In a week, she and her family were headed to Korea to spend time with her relatives, giving her a break from having cancer. She was worried that the pain would prevent her from enjoying the trip. Privately, she was worried about something a little sadder. I knew what was coming, but still, I was not ready to hear it. She began openly expressing her fears about the pain; the discovery of the new mass on her spine and several new metastases on her liver; how, if it were not for her son, she probably would have accepted her fate more gracefully, and not be fighting this hard to live. Her tears fell on her cheeks. We held hands across the table.

Six weeks had passed since that lunch date, Suzy had returned from Korea, and her pain had continued to increase. It was time to face the new problem head on. "Dr. J called today, but I didn't have the heart to call him back. I know what's ahead, but scared to hear him confirm it," this current text read when I was finally brave enough to open it.

I knew exactly how she felt. After my diagnosis, Dr. Jacobs' office had wanted to schedule my consult for the day after they discharged me from the hospital; I asked for a few extra days to grasp what was happening to me. In the same way, Suzy was not avoiding the news; she was just giving herself a few more normal days before the real work began.

Soon, she would meet with her oncology team to discuss the upcoming plan. Her new round of treatments would begin soon—this time her chemotherapy might be accompanied by radiation. I hoped with all my heart that she would not have to go through the full abdominal IMRT like I did. Imagining the effects of chemo on top of the horror that I went through with IMRT was too much to bear. How could anyone survive that? She did not deserve that level of suffering.

I had my next infusion of Avastin the following Tuesday, and with that came the hope of seeing Vicky. Someone else for me to worry about, as I had received no responses by email or text from her all week; it was not like her to be so silent. Her chemo must have been hitting her hard. Her treatment the previous week was canceled, so not hearing from her was giving me anxiety. I had two people who I loved, going through terrible effects of cancer and chemo, and all I could do was watch. I texted Vicky again that night, hoping this time she might answer and give an update on her situation.

Clearly, I was upset about something. Louis could see it in my face when I sat down next to him on the sofa for our nightly Netflix binge. I filled him in on Suzy's situation with the upcoming treatments, telling him what she had said to me at lunch all those weeks ago, while the tears rolled down my cheeks. "She's not ready to give in, so don't you give up on her," Louis said. I angrily swatted the tears from my face.

"I just don't get it," I said, getting control over myself. "Why did the drugs and radiation work so well for me, and yet, she's having all these problems?" Louis had no answer. "Why did those lesions on her liver grow despite twelve doses of chemo?" Louis shrugged. "And what the fuck is that thing on her spine?" Again, he had nothing.

I took a deep breath and tried to calm myself despite the rush of anger that was coursing through me. "Stupid fucking cancer. Fuck this shit. This is some actual bullshit." I was swearing wildly into the room. If profanity could cure Suzy's cancer, then I was Florence Fucking Nightingale.

There was no way around it. It was time to admit I felt guilty for my recent clear scan. Suzy had texted me the evening of my scan to find out the results and celebrated with me. And this is how she was rewarded for all her goodwill and friendship? She fought like hell to get through twelve doses of chemo this year, and now she gets to have another round *plus* radiation? Why do things continue to keep growing inside her? When would she get her big break? Suzy never feels sorry for herself, and what does it matter to cancer? I was going to feel indignant and angry on her behalf. I had a lot of rage bubbling up, and the skin of those bubbles was formed with guilt.

Eventually I calmed down. I would have to learn how to be a good friend to Suzy while not cultivating strange feelings about my own well-being.

One more blow to my delicate mental health was some news I had been dreading—a colleague of mine, a woman who had made food deliveries to me while I was going through chemo last year, had just told me her daughter-in-law, Jenn, had died from her cancer. Also in her 40s, Jenn was diagnosed with colon cancer six months before me. With a young child depending on her, she had tried every single treatment option available to her, including several clinical trials. The cancer continued to progress, and two years later, the end closed in fast; her airplane spiraled toward the ground. There would not be any last-minute rescue. After Jenn's death, it struck me just how brutally cold and unfeeling this predatory universe is. "There's no justice in this world," Dr. Kagan's words echoed yet again in my head. She was gone, and I was still here.

I struggled with the very real, overwhelming feelings of survivor's guilt. Even the privilege of naming the feelings I was having came with its own brand of guilt—having given myself an entitled excuse for justifying my present well-being. It would require a lot of hard work to navigate this very complicated emotion. Therapy was the only way I could cope; this was too big to do on my own.

Like onion layers, the awful truth slowly revealed itself, and I came to a conclusion that allowed me to breathe. The truth was the success of my treatments never depended upon nor reflected someone else's success. There was not a swap of lives to maintain some cosmic balance. There is no either/or option here. I am not permitted to live because someone else had to die in a one-to-one exchange. My success is completely unrelated to every other human being on this planet.

Is it luck? Is it karma? Is there something inherently different about my biology? Does it even matter? The answers to these questions will not change the fact that I am doing well right at this moment. Things could change, my cancer could reappear, but it was ok for me to be happy about my current health. As Traci had so aptly titled her book, I needed to remember that I was just one cancer patient in a sea of people.

Ta-Dah!

I didn't actually say, "Ta-dah!" but I was thinking it as I walked through the door into the rehearsal space.

It took many months to get to this moment, but it appeared as if I had worked through much of my trepidation about returning to performing. My cello case rolling noisily behind me, I trundled into the rehearsal room where half a dozen early arriving musicians were setting up their chairs and music stands. The orchestra would be crammed into this rehearsal space for the rest of the evening. I would be the only person wearing a surgical mask, but I was looking forward to making music again.

"Leeeeeee-saaaaaah!" Chuck is more to me than just the conductor of this orchestra; he is a friend. He was one of the very first people I met when I moved to Los Angeles in 2010. Several years ago, he rewrote the oboe concerto he had composed so that I could perform it with a flute choir accompanying me. It was a beautiful and haunting performance—bittersweet because it was the last concerto I would perform with my oboe before I had to put it down forever. He did not take this honor lightly, either.

Chuck is a big guy with a big personality who naturally commands attention and respect when he steps on the podium. And his heart is even bigger. Like a giant bear, he wrapped me up in his arms and squeezed me close. "I'm so glad you're here!" The last time I had seen him in person was almost six months ago, just after my reversal surgery. That day, I was very low on energy and incapable of socializing. On that occasion, he had hugged me more to hold me up. But this time I was squeezing back and laughing with joy.

"I should have asked if it was ok to hug you," he said, letting go. "Is it safe?" Because of my isolation all these months, I had forgotten just how small I am; he was towering over me.

"I have no idea." I smiled and shrugged. "And I don't care. All I know is life is too short to not hug my friends." He pulled me over for a friendly side-hug this time. You never know when it might be the last hug.

He tightened his grip for just a split second before adding, "I'm just so glad you're here."

He let me go and everyone else in the room took it in turns to greet and hug me, making it difficult to set up my chair and music stand. I could have spent the entire evening just doing this and never playing a single note. When I turned back, someone in the cello section had already set up my music stand for me.

There were a lot of nerves zinging around inside of me. It had been eighteen months since I last played my cello in public—a long time for a musician to go without performing. The COVID pandemic shutdown had forced all of us off the stage for nearly fifteen months. Crafty musicians found ways to perform together—mostly this involved experimentation with online conferencing programs, which made it impossible to play together in perfect sync thanks to the lag created by the video and audio processing software. The technology was great for companies who needed to hold morning meetings with employees working from home and for giving PowerPoint presentations. But it was terrible for live music. There were some music collaboration services that tried desperately to fill the gap in the market, but most of us quickly discovered that the software catered more to rock bands, not orchestras and classical musicians.

Many of us resorted to cutting up videos that made it appear as if we were performing together. An oboist who I have known since high school asked me to play some duets with her in this fashion. She recorded her part first, emailed the video to me, and then I recorded myself playing my cello along with her original video. She pieced the videos together, and the result was a fun video of her in her studio in Indiana, me in my yoga-slash-music room in California, miraculously playing duets together. It was fun, but still a letdown because we knew that this was not what making music *together* was about.

We broke the silence in the summer of 2021, when orchestras decided it was worth the risk to perform again. Our orchestra began giving outdoor concerts at a local park so that the audience and the musicians could count on a small amount of safety from the virus. There were several of us who still wore our masks, but many people were testing the waters and trying their luck without them during outdoor functions.

Those first rehearsals were exciting—people had not seen each other for over a year nor made music together in a live setting. There was so much catching up to do. Although the first few minutes were a little rough, the orchestra quickly adjusted to playing with each other again. We all resumed our usual professional demeanor as if no time had passed at all. During the lockdown, it felt as if things would never go back to normal, and yet, the moment the oboe played the tuning "A," everything that had happened during the previous year quickly became a distant memory.

The difference back then was that every single musician in the world was in the same position as me. Every person in the orchestra was wondering if they could play in tune? Would we remember how to read the conducting patterns? Did we still sound as good as before COVID? This time, I was the only person in the orchestra wondering about these things. All the musicians in this room had been playing together for more than a year and a half without me. They were back to their usual habits, so their expectations differed from mine now. If I made any stupid mistakes, everyone would hear me. Who else could it be? There was only one person in the orchestra who was rusty and out of practice.

While I was going through treatments, I spent a lot of time practicing my cello. The skin on my hands was peeling from the dreaded Hand and Foot Syndrome, but between chemo rounds, when my skin would heal a little, I spent as much time as I could scratching away on my cello. My friend Pam is also my cello instructor, and although we were not having formal lessons, she would send me texts now and again, "Why don't you start the 3rd movement of the Boccherini Concerto?" and "It's probably time to move on to the Popper 'Etude #10'." She would check on my progress, asking how things were going and if I needed any help with anything. But mostly giving me reassurance that as long as I was playing when I could, then I was going to maintain my skills. "The goal is to stay the same. Just don't let yourself slip and take steps backward!"

Yes ma'am!

Because of the Hand and Foot Syndrome, my calluses (the ones that build up on the tips of string players' fingers) were falling off. The new skin on my fingertips was soft and pink, burning and screaming every time I tried to play. But there is only one way to build up new calluses, and that is by playing, even if it meant playing through pain.

It was slow progress, but the little calluses *were* growing back. Maybe not as big or tough as they were before all this happened, but they were reappearing. My fingers were maintaining their strength and accuracy, my shoulders were strong and dependable, and despite my anxiety I could still read tenor clef. I just kept telling myself, "When this is over, I am going to be ready to get back to the stage." In my mind, there was no question about whether I would perform again, just as there had been no question about surviving cancer. I was working hard during treatments, expecting I would slip back into my former life without missing a beat.

There were so many starts and stops in my musical career—starting the flute when I was already an accomplished young pianist; once I was an advanced flutist, switching to the oboe and having to start from square one again; enjoying a solid career in New England, then packing up and starting over in Las Vegas; and, of course, moving from Las Vegas to Los Angeles, starting from scratch again only to have the devastating hernia that ended my oboe career. If I could go through all of that and have the moxie to start over again with the cello at 41, then I could get through cancer to come out the other side ready to work again. All I had to do was accept that, even now, I still had not reached a point in my life where I had career stability. I believed that only with that acceptance would I be able to move forward with confidence, grace, and optimism.

I would remind myself often: Cancer is so much worse than anything else happening to you. Just be patient with yourself. You can do this.

Sitting in the orchestra, which had already given four concerts in my absence, I looked around at my fellow musicians. According to the National Institute of Health (NIH), two in five Americans will have some type of cancer in their lifetime. Cancer math kicked—this meant roughly 25 of the musicians in this orchestra have had or will have some sort of cancer. I knew of more than a dozen people around me who had already survived cancer. But that only accounted for half of the statistic. After my diagnosis in 2021, three more members of the orchestra received their own cancer diagnoses. Just a few short weeks before this very rehearsal, one of those musicians was moved to hospice and passed away. Thinking of him cast a dark cloud over my joy as I saw a new face in his place and the empty seat where his widow, who had been taking time off to care for him and was now in mourning, usually sat. Again, I struggled with the eternal question of all cancer survivors: "What makes me so special that I survived and so many others don't?"

I knew many musicians (me included) were struggling with the difficulty of the piece. Long-time members had rushed home from work, eaten a quick dinner, and arrived to rehearsal on time; they were exhausted from a long day at work yet devoted to making music all evening. There were new people in the orchestra who were just getting to know their colleagues around them and trying to play their best. And then there was me, at the back of the cello section, hoping I could play well enough that my fellow cellos would not resent my return.

The first notes of Brahms' "Variations on a Theme by Haydn," which we were rehearsing, erupted from the orchestra. Despite the logistics of everyone's lives, those first notes were magnificent, glorious exaltations from Brahms—a man who long suffered from an unrequited love for another man's wife and toiled under the self-imposed artistic burden of believing he could never live up to the genius of Beethoven. I saw the piece as a fitting welcome for me—the simple theme was a reminder of my innocence in the Before Times; each variation increased in complexity, blurring the original melody. The piece reflected the way my life had become increasingly complex in the last eighteen months.

The notes coursed through my body, my cello vibrating in perfect symbiosis with the other instruments in the room, a physical manifestation of the ethereal dream of music. When he wrote these notes on the page, Brahms did not know 200 years later they would be the first notes a cancer survivor would play as she rejoined her life. Pen to paper on the cello line, he wrote the B-flat that would reverberate over the centuries to welcome me back. And bursting from my cello, it was the most joy filled note that I have ever played.

Of the 75 people making music that evening, I might have been the only one who had a spiritual experience. A thousand leaves glittering in the breeze, each note, from all the instruments, fluttering in my chest like butterflies awakening and erupting into the sky. The music was a joyful, colorful explosion of life. Nothing will ever be the same since cancer. And that, my friends, is the most wonderful gift of all.

Nesting

Despite what all my fancy photos on Instagram show, I actually have a tough time getting motivated to step onto my yoga mat and begin my practice each morning. I procrastinate in spectacularly complicated ways, often wasting half an hour just preparing to start my practice.

I begin by loading my teacher's YouTube channel, scrolling through all her videos, ignoring those with titles that promise backbends and king pigeon, finally settling on one that has a title I can live with like "Hip Stretches" or "Arm Balances and Inversions." While the video loads, I set up the room. Of course, I need to dig out the vacuum and go over the area rug (this is the only time I ever vacuum). While doing that, I will have noticed that I need to dust the windowsill (this is the only time I ever dust). Once the area rug is rolled up and tucked out of the way, it becomes clear I need to sweep the floor (this is the only time I ever sweep). When I unroll my yoga mat, there will be dirty paw prints on it, which, of course, I will need to clean off with the special cleansing wipes I have to spend five minutes looking for.

Once I am finally standing at the top of my mat, thumbs at my sternum, trying to get control over my breathing before I hit play on the video, I will notice the books and music in the bookcases need straightening; of course I need to take care of that before I begin. I will spend another ten minutes making sure all the spines line up perfectly straight. By that point, I usually have to pee or blow my nose or check on something the dogs are barking at in the backyard. It is a real testament to professional level procrastination.

The morning that I forced myself to skip the vacuuming, dusting, and all the extra moves was the morning I spotted my hummingbird friend once again in the tree branches just outside my window. Standing at the top of my mat, pleased with my ability to expedite the set-up process and stay focused this morning, I had just hit play on the video. My teacher was leading us through a breathing exercise when the little bird caught my eye. The video quickly and completely forgotten, I watched as a little green hummingbird flitted into view and then disappeared into the branches. I paused the video and stepped off my mat, moving closer to the window.

One of the unexpected side effects of chemo was the change in my vision. I have worn glasses pretty much my whole life—my fourth-grade teacher noticed I was squinting at the blackboard. After a phone call from the school, my parents whisked me off to the optometrist who fitted me for my first pair of glasses. In the seventh grade, feeling self-conscious as one of the few kids with glasses, I begged my mom to let me get contact lenses. From the age of 12 until I had cancer, I only wore contacts—though in my 40s reading glasses had to be added to the mix. Once I began chemo, my eyes were too dry for contacts; without eyelashes, I was fighting frequent eye infections; and eventually my eyesight worsened to where I needed two new prescriptions just three months apart. Now used to wearing my glasses all the time, I only wear my contacts for yoga or hiking. The trade-off is the vision correction is not as acute as with my glasses. I put up with it because it matters little while doing either activity.

This morning, I was cursing the contacts for making it difficult to see clearly what the hummingbird was doing. First, I squinted; then, I rubbed my eyes; briefly, my vision snapped into focus. If I avoided blinking, I could maintain this level of sight long enough to see what was going on in that tree.

I rubbed my eyes again, not because my vision was going out, but because I could not believe what I was seeing. The hummingbird was making another nest—maybe not in the exact same branch, but definitely in the same tree. There was a good chance that she was the same hummingbird whose nest I had watched the gardeners destroy in the story from *Round the Twist*. But did it matter if it was the same bird? The blatant coincidence of this unbelievable metaphor was good enough for me.

Like a dumbfounded cartoon character, my mouth was hanging open. If anyone had looked into my room, they would have thought I was frozen in time. By blinking again, my contacts could realign themselves, bringing the tiny bird and the invisible nest back into focus. The branch vibrated as she pieced together the new nest, and a slight chill ran down my neck. Tears stung my eyes, re-wetting the contacts, snapping the future tragedy into sharp focus.

"Crazy little bird. What are you doing?" I said out loud. I watched as she flew away, on the hunt for more spiderwebs with which to build her nest.

Obviously, she had forgotten what happened to her first nest in that very spot. Maybe that was for the best. Her naïveté might work to her advantage—someday. Against all odds, she was going to make her nest there. Maybe this year she would be successful.

My yoga practice abandoned, I stood by the window and watched her working on her new nest. I called Louis in—I wanted him to see what was going on, too. It was so difficult to see the tiny bird when she landed; she was so perfectly camouflaged amongst the leaves. "That's got to make you feel good," he said. "But what happened to doing yoga?" he ribbed, leaving the room to get back to work in his studio across the hall.

I knew I could not stand at the window and watch her forever, though it would be possible for me to keep an eye on her while doing yoga. I turned the video back on and resumed the breathing exercise. It was difficult to tear my eyes away from the nest building activities; it was fun to watch her throughout the hour while I was twisting into yoga shapes. Vowing this time to be much more vigilant against the gardeners, I made my plans for how best to protect this nest. I transmitted all the positive energy I could to the little bird, wishing her a more successful nesting season than the last time she used this tree. I was ready to do my part.

During practice this morning, the thrill of seeing my hummingbird friend reappear outside my window energized me. She was a gentle reminder that inspiration was all around me—tiny, camouflaged, fleeting messages hiding between the leaves of a bigger tree.

Her reappearance was as a harbinger, not an angel. She was not reinforcing my assumption that I needed to get back to the business of making music and trying to better my career. Building her nest once again on the ill-fated branch was not a sign that I should keep pursuing the same path I had been on before cancer. No matter how vigilant I might be, I already knew how her story was going to end—in a torrent of power tools and tears. She was showing me that doing the same thing over and over would always bring the same and expected outcome. If I changed nothing, then when I got back to work, I would continue for the rest of my life with the same result. I could fight this truth and repeatedly build my nest in the same branch—no matter how many times it is destroyed, I would persist and hope for a different outcome each time. Or I could accept this is how it will be, know the nest will be destroyed repeatedly—all the while, focusing parts of my attention and energies elsewhere. Some place more productive.

Since I spend so much time birdwatching, I learned hummingbirds build multiple nests during the nesting season. They literally do not put all their eggs in one basket. What was happening by my window was only one small aspect of the bird's attempt at raising a successful brood. There was no telling how many other nests she had built around the yard. Far from my watchful eye, she was stacking the deck in her own favor, building nests in several other trees, testing out which were the safest, out of the reach of clueless gardeners, and outside of my awareness.

The lesson to be learned from this bird was not about her futile persistence to rebuild in the same tree. The lesson was that she was keeping her options open, knowing full well that if one nest failed, one of her multiple back-ups might succeed.

I finished my yoga practice with another headstand. My view of the window flipped upside down, so now I was watching the bird flying inverted to the underside of the branch. Everything snapped into sharp alignment.

My hummingbird friend was absolutely right: I needed more nests.

Ha Ha, Fooled You

I spent more time trying to figure out what to name this chapter than I did writing the actual text of it. While reading another book, a potential title popped into my head. By the end of the paragraph, I had completely forgotten what it was. These sorts of memory lapses were a milder version of chemo brain. I thought that since more than a year had passed since my last dose of FOLFIRINOX, this would have ended. But, the nurses reminded me that Xeloda and Avastin are chemotherapy drugs. What I was experiencing at this point really was the same thing.

Somewhere in the neighborhood, there is a truck idling. For whatever reason, this is the most frightening sound in Dusty's world. I had been sitting at my computer in my yoga-slash-music room, toiling over the memory of this forgotten chapter title, when I heard his nails clicking on the terrazzo floor, growing louder as he approached my room. Moments later, he was standing next to my desk chair, his mouth open, lips curled back, panting like he had just run three miles at top speed to escape a monster. "What's the matter, Pooper?" I asked him. Sometimes I expect him to clear his throat and say, "The thing is, Mother Dear, I am terribly frightened of the truck and would really like your company right now." He may as well have said that; it was just as easy to read his eyes and furrowed brow.

Instead of stroking his fur and validating his fear, I tried something different. Grabbing his favorite blanket, a grey fleece which he constantly drags around my yoga-slash-music room floor, I made a cozy cave for him by piling it by my feet under my computer stand. He stood beside my chair for a few minutes, contemplating whether he should take his chance with this unfamiliar arrangement in exchange for being close to me while the scary truck continued to make noise. To my surprise, he took a few cautious steps into the dark desk-cave. I brought my feet up, sitting cross-legged on the chair, giving him more space. The delight I felt when he finally laid down on the blanket and rested his head on his paws was overwhelming. Seeing this as an opportunity to take a break from the blank page on my screen and the panicky dog by my feet, I checked my email. My delight deflated almost instantly.

I had a feeling that the insurance company's silence all these months was too good to be true. It appeared they had decided today was the day when the bills would begin rolling in from this year's chemotherapy treatments. I had once tried to calculate the cost of all my FOLFIRINOX treatments, but it was so confusing to piece together all the separate charges listed in my hospital portal, and nearly impossible for me to remember the names of all nine drugs and the various medical equipment involved in the infusions. I reached a point where I no longer cared about what they were charging—rather *over*charging—the insurance company for services. What was more concerning was that I had not yet seen any bills toward my insurance deductible since January. Many months had passed, and it was pointless to hope the hospital simply forgot to bill me.

The bills were there now, just sitting there waiting for me in my hospital portal (exactly as the email had proudly announced). The best part was, with just three quick and painful payments, I would pay the deductible off. Even after all I have been through with cancer, I still suffered from financial resentment for paying necessary expenses like taxes, insurance premiums, or, in this case, medical bills. This amounted to a general feeling of panic, but also of not wanting to waste our money on this stuff. All these months later, my insurance still had not approved the treatments for osteoporosis—I was frozen on the bottom step of the infamous "Step Therapy" practice, unable to move forward even though I had already failed on a lesser drug.

As I clicked "Pay Now" on the payment portal, I reminded myself this was a heck of a lot better than not having insurance at all. We are both self-employed musicians. Without the Affordable Care Act, I would never have been approved for private insurance to pay for my care—in the two years since my diagnosis, my medical bills easily added up to more than $2 million. Who knows how much more my care would cost before this was all over? It would bankrupt us. Still, I rolled my eyes and *tsk'd* and *sighed* as if I had a choice in the matter. What a magnificent house we could buy with two million dollars in cash!

In the meantime, soul-searching about my career was in full swing. I had made it through my first rehearsal in one piece, but instead of spending hours practicing my cello, I was sitting at my computer typing. I was editing the manuscripts of other authors, which I enjoyed. They happily overlooked the fact that I am utterly unqualified to do that work; I assumed they were just being polite in asking me to do this. Perhaps because I had a book picked up by a real publisher, they thought I had talent and sudden expertise. But I felt like a fraud correcting their formatting issues, removing extra spaces after periods, catching all the spelling and grammatical errors they had become blind to, eliminating contractions with creative alternatives, and rewriting awkward passages. I wrote professional sounding blurbs and reviews and provided rough drafts of the back of the book summaries for them. Maybe I had some actual talent for writing and editing, even though I had no training in the field. I enjoyed the work and began actively seeking more projects with other authors.

Obviously, I could never give up being a musician. But I was interested in giving up the habit of not earning a living. Louis kept us comfortable, which meant I never had to work. I simply wanted to work because I wanted to work. Because my career had come to a full stop when I started from scratch on the cello in my 40s, I could not go the traditional music career route: graduate from college, take some auditions, win some auditions, and then work my way up the musical ladder, someday landing a permanent, well-paying, orchestral job. Even if I had never had cancer, at 49, there still is not enough time to accomplish everything I wanted to with the cello. By the time I reached the important milestones, I would already be too old.

Since cancer had given me the opportunity to reevaluate my life, I felt it was time to accept that maybe the traditional path was never in my future, anyway. Instead of fighting against it, maybe it was time to embrace the multiple paths laid out before me. What if I did not have to pick just one and stick with it? What if I had options? My mind turned back to the hummingbird with her multiple nests.

Round the Twist was a labor of love. Most people write their cancer memoirs long after they have finished treatments. Reflecting on their experience years later, they feel a desire to share after they are in remission. They compile their stories from notes, journals, memories, and interviews. Not me. I wrote the book in real time. I had the audacity to imagine that I was writing a book while I was writing a book. It was fun to give the chapters quirky titles and to compose provocative closing sentences. I said writer-type things around the house like, "I'm going to spend the afternoon working on my book," and Louis encouraged me. I wrote for hours upon hours, documenting my experience as it was happening. I was not squinting into a hazy past obscured by a cloud of drugs and fear. I had put it all there on the page in real time. A year later, after the heavy drugs wore off, I would read my own words and be shocked by how much of it I did not remember writing. I was thankful for this portal into my past—those memories now only existed on the page, not in my head. It seemed like I might have created something unique.

I belong to a Facebook group for the writers signed by my publisher. I felt like a phony when I posted for the first time, "Thrilled to have signed my first book contract with Black Rose Writing. Thanks for having me!" Within an hour, there were over twenty comments of "Welcome!" And "Can't wait to read your book!" A few of the authors offered to read my manuscript and write reviews. Every day, people posted questions about marketing, sales tax, editing software, cover design, review swaps, and author events. The other writers posted funny memes, and I was shocked to find out I was enough "in the know" to get the inside jokes. Beyond that, I was making friends who I wanted to spend time with, whose opinions I respected, and who seemed to accept me into their circle. I had found my kin.

One morning, an author posted the question: "How do you spend your time between your final draft submission and launch?" The first and only answer posted to this question was dry and to the point: "Write your next book."

I stopped in my tracks. My next book? Even though it was not meant for me, the comment struck a chord. *Round the Twist* ended with me leaving the hospital after my colostomy reversal and the surgeon's declaration, "No visible sign of disease." Artistically speaking, this was the right place to end the book. I would not go into the details of my adjuvant therapy, my sexual dysfunction, or my simmering PTSD. There were 25,000 words beyond the last line of the book, "It was time to play in the grass again," sitting on my computer, though. When I submitted the manuscript for consideration, in November 2022, I cut out and pasted those additional chapters into a new Word document, titled it "Part 2," and threw it into a folder on my desktop that had the audacious label: "Books." No one can ever accuse me of not dreaming big.

What I would do with "Part 2" remained to be seen. The idea of writing about the daily doldrums of my post-cancer life made my head feel dull. Who would be interested in hearing about this part? Things were going back to normal. What could be interesting about Lisa-without-cancer? Did people really want to read about me doing yoga, practicing my cello, and freaking out about scans? A book about me growing my hair back promised to be about as interesting as a TED Talk on the stages of drying paint.

After signing my contract for *Round the Twist*, I set to work polishing every surface until that thing shined. Now it was time to fill out the story, to add more details (which Louis provided since his memory was not affected by the hardcore chemotherapy drugs), expand on certain topics, and provide even more stories. As I recalled events for him to corroborate, I thought I had a handle on the timeline and validity of the memories. Turned out, my memory sucked—I remembered almost nothing of the weeks I was on chemo. Together, we put together a timeline of my spotty memories and his hard facts. Without this clarification, I could never have created the chapters documenting those twelve weeks. Three editors worked on the book, tightening up the story timeline and giving me homework to rewrite sections and even whole chapters. Early reviewers sent blurbs which made it sound like an actual writer wrote the book. For the first time, I realized I had created something worth sharing and I might not be an imposter after all.

The beautiful cover (a team effort between the publisher's graphics team, and my artist uncle who painted the original image) hit my inbox four months before launch, and I was excited to post it on my website, to plaster it on newsletter blasts, and to flood my Facebook Author Page with it. I imagined the book in bookstore displays and saw myself holding it up while standing in front of eager readers. Between editing deadlines and PDF galleys, I was sitting down at the computer every afternoon to write. I typed about the daily things happening to me and gave voice to thoughts that were bouncing around in my head. "Just get it out and worry about what to do with it later," a fellow writer had advised me when I told her I was not sure this second project was worth it. Like my new friend advised, I stopped caring about what I was writing, and just got it out of my head. Before I knew it, I had 60,000 words, yet only a vague idea of what this book was about.

At the end of concerts, when the orchestra is standing for bows, my fellow oboist, Bob, would say to me under the applause, "Welp, fooled 'em again!" The first time he said it, I laughed. But, I started thinking it to myself after every concert from that point forward. And long after I stopped playing oboe, waving to Bob from my new seat in the cello section, I imagined him saying it to the new oboist. Ever since, I have made a point of saying it to whoever is closest to me on every stage, thanks to him.

This feels exactly like what I have done with writing. Maybe I should have ended the book with "Ha-ha, fooled you!" as the last line.

Taking a step back, I could see the overall picture. What to name the book seemed obvious—*Welcome to the Bright*—after the last chapter of *Round the Twist*. On the surface, it is a positive and sunny description. But with a deeper understanding, it aptly describes how it feels to suddenly be thrust out into the world after cancer. Like a newborn, everything is overwhelming—the sights, the sounds, the sunlight. The glare off the world is blinding. Everything feels exaggerated and sometimes even painful. The slightest emotion quickly runs out of control, so I shield my eyes from the sight of bright hope.

Welcome to the Bright was simply a collection of musings about my life after cancer. I was exploring the topics I wanted to read about at this stage in my recovery, yet could not find the resources. I was creating my own survivor handbook. So, I stopped being so critical of myself. I was not fooling anyone. I was simply trying to address the elephant in the room: what happens to us when the treatments are over?

Very few survivors talk about this phase. Very few people around us stop to consider its existence. This means there is very little information out there for any of us. Alone as I navigated these waters, I mostly relied on Ella and Alice to help me paddle my little kayak through the unexpected rapids. How many people are lucky enough to have an Ella or Alice by their side through this part?

In the six months between signing my contract and finishing the final manuscript, I probably read *Round the Twist* over 100 times. Nearly every word memorized, I knew each turn in the story by heart. My head was a whirlpool swirling with my prose, threatening to suck me to the bottom of a deep, emotional ocean. The result was that I was becoming depressed having to relive chemo, radiation, surgery, the colostomy, and all the stress of cancer, repeatedly for long hours every day. I would finish a chapter and weep at my desk, dreading what happens on the next page. I had to build a barrier between the raw emotions and the words on the page. It took a while, but I learned to read the work from an objective point of view, protecting my delicate heart from reliving the events with vicious sadness. And all the while, working on *Welcome to the Bright* gave me some relief. It brought me back to the present, a difficult present to be sure, but the only one in which I belonged.

Is this book my public therapy or is it the universal theme of cancer survival? Did millions of people share my experience with recovering, coping with the aftermath of cancer, and trying to live their fullest life? Probably yes, no matter how alone I felt.

"No one ever talks about this part," Ella confirmed. I had just admitted I did not feel ready to get back on stage despite having attended the first rehearsal. She grew quiet across the table, taking a sip of the Central Coast Cabernet she had indulged in at our lunch. "It's hard to articulate why we have trouble getting back to our normal lives. People want us to just go back to the way we were, because *they* want this to be over. They're tired of *you* having cancer. The truth is, we never live up to their expectations."

Pam has been very sensitive and thoughtful with me. Although she was eager to get me back in the orchestra, she was one of the few people who had watched my initial decline happen in real time, living every scary moment with me up to my diagnosis. Because of that, she understands why I am still frightened and sometimes cry in the middle of a sentence for no obvious reason. She sees I am not the same, so she does not treat me the same. She has become patient with me, though sometimes she has trouble containing her enthusiasm for how I am doing. "I'm so proud of you!" she exclaimed during my first lesson in over six months. I became flustered and even got a little teary-eyed. She mercifully pretended not to have noticed, and moved on with the lesson, not forcing me to put into words the reason for my emotional reaction.

Lori is so far away, she can only check on me with calls, texts, and emails. And yet, she never asks the trite question, "How are you?" She already knows how I am. Instead, Lori reminds me how much she loves me, and Alice tells me she is there if I need anything. Neither ever say the words, "Don't worry, everything is going to be ok." Because they know nothing is going to be ok ever again. And how could anyone assume to know what lies in my future? Instead, both encourage me to visit them in New York when I am a famous author appearing on the *Today Show*, talking about my book. They make me smile and laugh and remind me to never underestimate what I can do.

Through writing, I have learned to say, "I *had* cancer." Thanks to the process of organizing the book, I could start thinking more seriously about how I might want to organize myself.

To get the heaviness of so many reads of *Round the Twist* off my shoulders, I plowed through the *Harry Potter* series, enjoying the simple pleasure of the literary equivalent of licking the frosting off a cupcake. I downloaded books by authors interviewed on NPR and devoured them in days. I sang along to loud music in the car as I drove around on errands and took pictures of ridiculous things like my dogs laying in the dirt in the backyard.

What gave me a true sense of purpose was doing what I could to take care of my friends. Knitting caps and bringing food to Vicky felt like I was helping, even if there was really nothing I could do. For all her strength and positivity, she was struggling with the late stages of her cancer. During my most recent visit, she was coughing up blood. And yet, when she had settled back against her pillow, she squeezed my hand and soothed me with her warm smile, "This too shall pass." She was facing her oncoming fate with stoic grace. I could take advantage of my current good health and be the one standing on solid ground. I was holding on to Vicky with all my strength. My heart would not be the only one to break when she inevitably slipped over the edge.

Today, I stopped by to drop off some warm bread for Suzy. She burst into tears on my shoulder in her front yard. "No one really understands how amazing all this is," she said when she finally loosened her grip on the back of my shirt. She motioned toward the grass at our feet. I wiped a tear from her cheek.

We hugged one more time. I placed my hand on the small of her back, beneath which lay the new and troublesome cancerous tumor along her spine, while her hand found its way into my growing hair, twisting her fingers into the longer strands. Holding on to each other under the glorious blue sky, we could cure the cancer in our bodies, the cancer in our minds, and stand forever on the miraculous grass growing beneath our feet.

The Burial

"Someone riddled with cancer doesn't have the amount of energy that you do," Alice's declaration continued to bounce around inside my head. It had been nearly a year since she first spoke those words to me over the phone; they were just as important now as they had been last spring.

More than half a year had passed since Dr. Quilici told me there were no visible signs of disease inside my body. I was no closer to accepting this than I was that day. All that had changed was my physical state. I was strong. I was healthy. I was energetic. I was healing.

Deep in the weeds of chemo, I was frustrated at how the drugs and the disease had clobbered my body. "This is all temporary," I would remind myself. "One year from now, this will all be a distant memory." Statistically[3], it was more likely I would be dead in a year, and *Lisa* would be the distant memory.

The theoretical year after chemo had passed, and my recovery was inarguably miraculous. Ignorant of the harsh truth of my prognosis, I never doubted that I would make a full recovery. And my recovery seemed to be going well. Yet, I was hiding out in my house as if I were still on the drugs, just as delicate and breakable as I was then. I was acting as if I had pain, fresh stitches, and healing tissue. These things now only existed in my head, like wet nail polish.

---

[3] In 2024, Stage-4 CRC has a 5-year survival rate of 13%

Going to my appointments at Dr. Jacobs' office at the Disney Cancer Center, I felt exposed, leaving the safety of my car to walk through the parking garage and along the sidewalk to the main entrance. I wore my mask, even though I was outside and there were no people anywhere near me. Swirling around me were invisible, deadly microbes in the air sure to infiltrate my weak immune system and kill me. The rest of the world was acting like there was nothing to be afraid of. I was seeing clouds of germs, puddles of bacteria, and swarms of viruses in shocking technicolor. Danger lurked everywhere; the air filling my lungs was a deadly poison. I was turning into a paranoid germaphobe.

Occasionally, Louis and I would stop at the health foods market to pick up something fun for lunch after my appointments. As the only people in the store wearing masks, we got sideways glances from the other customers. Although they did not voice their criticism, they certainly made no attempt to hide their disdain for my continued mask wearing. Joking with Louis in the snack aisle, I said, "maybe I should shave my head again so people will leave me alone." I only knew how to move through the world with a mask and a bald head; baldness appears to be the universally accepted sign of a dire health condition, and not to be questioned.

I was still clinging to certain daily routines I had adopted during chemo and radiation, none of which were tied to the clock, and none which might lead to any semblance of productivity—yoga in the morning, practicing my cello all afternoon, and finishing out the evening with Louis on the sofa surfing through Netflix until bed.

I had taken the plunge by attending my first rehearsal despite my self-doubt. Just as I had feared, most people at rehearsal were not wearing a mask, and yet I had survived. My body was doing just fine, and I played well. To the outside observer, my return to rehearsals was a success. But my mind was still stuck in its protective bubble. I was still anxious about getting together with friends. Even if I enthusiastically accepted an invitation, I would spend the hours ahead of our date filled with anxiety, debating whether to cancel on them. Social anxiety was festering within me and I was developing an unhealthy obsession with staying healthy. Not a good combination.

The oncology team had recently added a new condition to my medical records—*persistent immunodeficiency secondary to chemotherapy*. Not only did I have untreated osteoporosis, but my bone marrow was still struggling to recover from all the treatments I had been through. This did not necessarily turn me into a porcelain doll. Dr. Jacobs said it was time to get back out there. He had given me a clear prescription; I just needed to cowgirl up and swallow the giant horse pill.

My friends and colleagues knew that the scary treatments were over. They knew that I had had clear scans, and the doctors had told me I was *technically* disease free. Everyone expected me to jump at the chance to get out of the house, to go to all the places I had been avoiding for the past year, and to get back to doing the things that made me who I am. Friends would call, hoping to catch up with a simple conversation on a lazy Saturday, and I would let the call go to voicemail. They had no idea what was going on inside of me.

Ella understood why I was hesitating to join in on real life. "You'll know when it's time to get back out there. There's no need to rush yourself just to make other people happy." Perhaps she was right. But there was a thin line between taking my time and cowering. A new cancer had infiltrated my mind—it would take more than a little chemo and radiation to kill this variety.

The furniture in my yoga-slash-music room is all lined up against the walls, leaving the center completely open for me to do yoga or practice my cello. In fact, there is so much floor space that sometimes Louis can unroll his mat next to mine and join me for a yoga session, the furniture completely out of our way.

The room is underutilized, but I refuse to give up the wide-open space.

Along one wall, I have a row of bookcases which house all my sheet music. It would be impossible to count how much music I have collected in the past 30 years—by my estimate, I have over 1000 pieces of music in my library. Under the window, my two cellos sit quietly on their stands, the bows stored on the wall shelves my father made for me a few years earlier when I was setting up my room. Since this is a spare bedroom I am using as my office, there is a closet jam-packed with various instrument cases, photo albums, boxes of forgotten DVDs, and Andrew's graduation cap and gown. The fourth wall is blank, except for two hanging yoga rugs. I practice all the upside-down poses near this wall, so if I fall, I have the wall to catch me. After 25 years of yoga, I hardly ever use the wall. But I like to keep the option open. You know, just in case.

My computer had been on a rolling stand since I moved into this room two years ago—I tuck it into the closet between the cello case and the vacuum, wheeling it out when I feel inspired to write, or when I join a Zoom meeting. This never bothered me, but Louis could hardly stand this set up. Every time he would walk by my room, seeing me working or writing on this little computer stand pushed up against the closed closet door, he would stop. Standing in the doorway, he would offer his opinion. "We need to get you a proper desk," he would say. Naturally, his eyes land on the blank wall, where my yoga rugs hang. "And it could go right there."

"Nope," I would shake my head. "That's where I do my handstands."

"Can't you do handstands against the closet door?" He had a point. That was probably a more sensible place to practice those. But he knows I would never willingly grant him the satisfaction of being right.

Conversation over. For now, nothing would disrupt my yoga-slash-music room's setup.

And yet, he had been successful in planting a seed—I mulled over the possibilities for several days. Eventually, I became restless. "If I were to put a desk somewhere, and it wasn't against my blank wall, where would it go?" I asked Louis as he, once again, stood in my doorway trying to convince me of the change.

His suggestion was to upend one bookcase, making some space for a desk between it and the other bookcase, which would remain horizontal. It took me a few more days to wrap my brain around the change, but I finally got there. One morning, when I was supposed to be practicing yoga, I pulled out nearly 500 pieces of music from one bookcase, stacked them on the floor, and hoisted the entire piece of furniture up to vertical on my own. The next time Louis passed by my doorway, he stopped, this time out of surprise. "You should have called for me to help you lift that!" I wonder what Dr. Jacobs would think about me moving heavy furniture around by myself?

Once I get an idea in my head, nothing can stop me. Now, all we needed was to buy a desk to fit the space. A quick order on Wayfair, and the desk would arrive in 5-7 business days. Although at first resistant to changing my room, now I was excited for the fresh start. My nest was getting an update.

While I was moving my yoga altar during the big move, I came face to face with the sodalite stone and amethyst Ganesh statue that I had clutched throughout chemo. They rested on a small ceramic dish with a snake painted on it. After chemo, I never ever touched these stones again. I stood for quite some time staring at them, and all the broken bits, before carefully lifting the dish and replacing it on the other bookcase, making sure nothing spilled during the transfer.

I was not afraid of the stones, but I felt a real disdain and revulsion toward them. All I knew was that under no circumstance should I touch them with my bare skin. They contained the energy of the cancer that had been removed from my body during my treatments last winter. Maybe it sounded crazy, but I felt I needed to be cautious around them.

When dealing with healing stones, there is a ritual of burying them in the Earth to rid ourselves of them. This is done to allow the planet to absorb and safely disperse the harmful energies contained within. Almost a year ago, I had decided I would bury the stones up on the mountain, somewhere off the hiking trail, when I was ready. Would I know when was the right time to do this thing?

It had been raining nearly nonstop for several weeks this spring. In Southern California, this is unheard of. This is the most rain I have ever seen in my thirteen years here. Sinkholes were opening in the roads in our little corner of the valley, water was rushing rivers through the streets into the drainage ditches, and our backyard was a muddy mess in which the dogs were having a grand time playing. Desperate to get out of the house, I wasted no time in hitting the hiking trails after the rain stopped.

It was a Saturday morning like any other. I awoke just as the sun was coming up. And as usual, I was trying to lie perfectly still and quiet so the dogs would not hear me and try to dig me out from under the blankets until I was ready to face my day. My mind snapped to the stones. Today I do it.

While the morning sun burned off the May Gray, I dressed for the hike, found a gardening trowel in the garage, and stuffed it in my daypack. I tipped the two stones, and the chipped amethyst pieces, into a small plastic zipper bag. I donned my gaiters and *fuck cancer* baseball cap, slipping out the door before the dogs realized I was leaving them behind.

Not knowing where I was going to bury the stones, I spent the half-mile walk to the park trying to visualize the trails and the mountain. Maybe by the time I got there, I would know where to bury them. They would need to be buried in a place I did not pass often. I wanted the cancer energy they contained to be hidden and inaccessible to me forever. It may have been too much to hope for, but I wanted to forget the place, so I would never be tempted to look for them in the future.

The ground was wet and muddy in places, and there were mini landslides along the trail—rocks the size of softballs had tumbled into the path, making one of my favorite trails difficult, and nearly impossible, to navigate. Distracted by the obstacles in the trail and the reinvention of the landscape, I quickly forgot the stones in my pack. Enjoying the paradox of the warm sun on my face and the cool air licking the exposed skin on the back of my neck, I was surrounded by sound—squawking crows and screeching hawks playing on the thermals above me, and a dog barking somewhere on one of the lower trails. With the rolling landscape between us, the distant horn of a train passing through the tunnel on the north side of the park was faint by the time it reached me. I hiked for nearly an hour, lost in the exotic beauty of the rain-changed familiar landscape around me. Deep within the hills, I could no longer see the valley below; all signs of civilization obscured by nature. Looking out at the wild hills, I could breathe again.

My feet stopped moving, as if they had a mind of their own. A strange sensation crept through my chest, a little warm, somewhat giddy. I looked to my left—I squinted at the mountain rising into the morning sun; to my right was yet another hill with several large boulders lying at its feet. One, the size of a school bus, caught my eye amongst a few scraggly desert trees. This was it: the spot I would bury the crystals to be forgotten forever.

The boulder was about 200 feet off the trail. I would need to tramp through the tall grasses to reach it. My mind conjured up hidden rattlesnakes; I was certain there were hundreds of them between where I stood on the trail and the boulder. Then again, if I was meant to bury the stones there, surely the Earth would clear the path. I had my trekking poles in hand, so with each step, I used them to disturb the tall grasses ahead of me. Imaginary snakes were the least of my worries. I should have been more concerned about the very real roots, rocks, and muddy patches that threatened to twist my ankle. Remembering my untreated osteoporosis, I slowed my pace and took more care with each step.

Reaching the boulder, I propped my trekking poles against a bush beside me and sat down with my back against the giant rock. Hiking always makes my hands and fingers swell, which makes it difficult to do anything that requires fine motor control—like unzipping my pack. This morning, there was no rush. So what if it took me ten minutes to get the zipper open? I took out the trowel and began digging into the spongy earth. The heavy rains had saturated the usually rock solid, cement-like earth. The soft ground was easy to break apart so I could bore a perfect hole for my crystals. I dug down as deep as I could before hitting too many roots and stones, preventing me from digging any further. Turning my eyes upward, I thanked the skies for the rain.

Setting aside the trowel, I reached into my pack and found the small baggie with the stones in it. While I had these stones with me, I felt comforted and strong, and they gave me courage while facing chemo and radiation. In a few moments, the stones, and the cancer contained within, would be buried deep in the damp earth—the unmarked grave where they would rest until the end of time.

Holding up the baggie, I pondered over the stones, my mind filled with questions. Do I thank them for absorbing the cancer? Do I thank them for bringing me comfort? Do I say goodbye? Should I say nothing and just dump them in the hole because fuck cancer? I stared at them for several minutes, marveling at what I believed they had done for me. I unsealed the baggie and prepared to tip them into the hole.

My hand hesitated. I wanted to keep them. I loved these stones. They represented the darkest months of my life. How could I just discard and abandon them? They were so beautiful, and the way the sunlight was glinting off them was mesmerizing—only now, in the bright sunlight, did I appreciate the exquisite details in the grains of the amethyst. The stones were making their last appeal to stay their execution. This was crazy; I should just keep them.

A voice spoke up inside of me. "You need to get rid of these stones and the cancer if you ever want to move on with your life."

I closed my eyes and took a deep breath. "Don't hold on to this," I said out loud. "You have to let it all go." I waited, feeling the anxiety move through me as a jolt of adrenaline. I visualized it flowing out through the top of my head, disbursing into the clouds above me, and down through my feet, like roots in the earth. Taking another deep breath, and slowly exhaling through slightly parted lips, I whispered, "I am letting you go," and tipped the baggie's contents into the hole.

The little voice inside of me rejoiced, "They're gone!" I stuffed the empty baggie in my backpack and picked up the trowel, plunging it into the pile of displaced earth next to the hole. My hand and arm were paralyzed. I could take the crystals out of the hole and bring them back home where they belong. It was not too late.

"No!" I spoke aloud. "Lisa, for fuck's sake, let them go!" Anyone passing by on the trail would have thought I was having a mental break right there in the wilderness.

Before I could change my mind yet again, I scooped the dirt into the hole, imagining the sunshine being blotted out from their point of view. I disturbed the grasses and roots nearby to hide my handiwork, collected my poles, and stood up. The hills around me seemed somehow brighter, friendlier, and a little wilder. Had this place always been this beautiful? This time, when I breathed in deep and exhaled, it was with laughter.

The stones, and the cancer, were gone.

Detour

The son of a friend of ours was diagnosed with cancer at 7. After a horrible year of treatments, they gave him his clean bill of health, and he is now just like any normal 11-year-old boy. Our friend told me she never liked the term Post Traumatic Stress Disorder. She preferred to call it PTS. "It's not that you're having a disordered reaction to a normal situation. You're having the expected reactions to an outrageously abnormal situation."

There was nothing normal about having cancer. There was nothing normal about chemotherapy or radiation. There was nothing normal about sleeping in my bed with a small pump lying next to me that injected me with a powerful drug every 90 seconds. There was nothing normal about losing almost a foot of my colon or having a colostomy. There was nothing normal about dropping 18 pounds or losing my hair. There was nothing normal about any of this. I have emotional scars. People either need to accept this new version of me, or they need to move on.

Why should anyone try to convince me that the reactions I was having, the feelings I was feeling, were inappropriate and needed to be fixed? After going through a traumatic experience, why are we expected to conform to what other people consider normal? Instead, we should agree that from this point on, our normal—every cancer survivor's normal—is going to be different from those around us. We need to accept that this is not only ok, but to be embraced. No one needs to fix me; I am wonderful the way I am now.

While I was going through active cancer treatments, people found it difficult to see me crying, or hurting, or complaining—maybe they wanted this to be over for their own personal reasons. Perhaps they are not equipped to witness someone else going through an emotional experience. Some tried out platitudes on me like "Everything happens for a reason." They believe it's helpful, but mostly it feels like a hint that they felt it was time for me to get over it. I came to believe I was the problem—I was the one feeling the wrong things, and it was my fault they felt uncomfortable. It took me a long time to understand that it might have little to do with them wanting me to feel better, and more to do with their desire to avoid figuring out how to cope with me. Slowly, I understood that it was on them to make themselves feel better. If they were having a difficult time accepting the way I was behaving, then that was on them. It was not my responsibility to soothe them. They needed to figure this out for themselves, and not expect me to do it for them.

These post-cancer months were going to be filled with these sorts of realizations. Working on my PTSD was going to be a solo journey to discover my new normal. This had nothing to do with any other person on the planet and their comfort.

I have great difficulty in looking at photos of myself from before my diagnosis—like looking at a stranger, or a distant aunt who died when I was a kid. I hardly recognize my former self. Now, an alien masquerading as something familiar mimics me the best they can. I had hoped to come through this thing as a better version of myself. Now I worried I would be this panicky mess forever. What I needed from my friends was support, not pressure to return to the way I was before; they needed to tell me they loved me even in this new messy form. Maybe New Lisa struggles with being in crowds, and New Lisa wants more private time. Maybe New Lisa feels nauseous when she smells peppers cooking, but New Lisa also discovered that she feels no guilt about eating ice cream for breakfast.

Around the 1-year post-chemo mark, the nurses and doctors started asking very specific questions about my mental health. Was I sleeping well? Did I have nightmares? How were my appetite and activity levels? Was I feeling any stress or anxiety? But most importantly, how was I coping in the aftermath of cancer? They could not have been more point blank with their queries, and Abby, now giving me my Avastin infusions every three weeks, was sitting in my cubicle with me and talking frankly about what I should expect from myself.

I hardly think the dreams I was having could be called nightmares—I knew what those were like, I'd had my fair share of wake-up-screaming nightmares since my diagnosis. These days, I sometimes dreamt of giant machines, and diagnoses of new cancers, or of waking up during a surgery—I would awaken in my bed disoriented, believing I was in a hospital room. But I was also having vivid dreams about swimming with dolphins and riding horses, from which I would wake up still feeling their warmth and fur against my body, leaving me filled with joy and hope.

I had changed many of the sound notifications on my iPhone so that they did not resemble electrical beeps and avoided certain chairs in Dr. Jacobs' waiting room—I did these things without stopping to consider why. Shortly after I finished radiation, my mouth would get dry as we approached the freeway exit for the hospital, I got shaky when I heard the parking ticket being printed in the meter machine at the entrance to the parking garage, and the sound of the elevator doors made my knees weak. I needed to work through these things on my own schedule—I didn't need someone to fix me. With time and effort, I might learn to avoid the triggers, and avoid some of the reactions. Though it would never change the fact that something horrible happened to me in that building. It was up to me, on my own timeline, to make my peace with myself.

During a dramatic temper tantrum, I threw out the shirts that I wore during chemo and radiation; I avoided the clothing I wore to accommodate my colostomy bag, tucking certain yoga pants into the back of the drawer. These things did not add up. I did not see what was happening—it was Ella and Alice who brought the truth behind these behaviors to my attention.

The most obvious symptom was my hesitance to perform in a concert. I thought by beginning there, forcing myself to attend one rehearsal and taking that first step, I could just coast along until I was better. The old *fake it 'til you make it* chestnut. My first rehearsal back with the orchestra had felt like a colossal success.

The problem was each rehearsal that followed. Driving to the second rehearsal, my heart was pounding; I was dreading more hugs from the other musicians. I desperately wanted to be normal again, to set up my music stand and tune my cello in anonymity like in the Before Times. I wanted to stop feeling the eyes of the other musicians scanning me while I played. I understood why they did it—I would do it, too, if one of my colleagues had also peered into the eyes of Death and returned a year later looking scrawny and beat up.

Carefully planning my arrival this time, most people didn't even notice me walking into the rehearsal room, so I was able to take my seat and hide in plain sight without anyone loudly announcing my arrival. Only the other cellists around me would greet me. Judy, a violinist I had played with in this orchestra for years, was waving discreetly at me through the gaps in the musicians seated between us. Seeing her smile at me, knowing that she had also been through this exact process over a decade ago, gave me the confidence that I was not unique or treading aimlessly in unchartered waters. Her look was not sympathetic or pitying; she was welcoming me back to the real world where we were survivors floating within a sea of regular people.

Pam, being our principal cellist, sits directly in front of me. She had driven me to several radiation treatments, had brought us lunch and visited with me during chemo, and she had been my constant cheerleader—much of this accomplished while she was recovering from major spine surgery. As we ate lunch together on my patio shortly after my diagnosis, she said to me, "Obviously I have no idea what you're going through, but I'm here however you need me." She took the time to watch, listen, and learn. She discovered that cancer patients are both delicate and fierce. She showed the world that if you do not close your eyes while your friend goes through the scary stuff, you will witness something incredible. It often felt as if very few people wanted to see these changes happening to me. But she did—she both embraced and encouraged them. And now, just her presence during these critical first steps was giving me the confidence to be at these rehearsals. The back of her head became my anchor and lifeline.

Bow to string, the rehearsal began, and I was glad to be caught up in the energy of the orchestra again. But very quickly, it became clear that the overwhelming volume of the ensemble was short-circuiting my brain. The hands on the clock moved slowly, and a flutter was growing in my belly. The music on my stand swam in front of my eyes—it felt as if I had never been able to read music. I forgot how to hold the bow, and my fingers groped for the proper strings. I put my arms down and took a deep breath. My throat tightened, and I found it impossible to swallow. *You're choking!* a voice in my mind screamed. Pam's head continued to sway with the music. Her performance was driven and confident. As her bow dug into the strings, deep accents made certain notes stick out from the long melodic line, while her body moved with the strength and assuredness brought on by a lifetime of making music.

I breathed in through my nose and out through my mouth. I tried unsuccessfully to swallow again; my heart raced. Was it possible that I was *actually* choking? My stand partner took one quick sideways glance at me, but then had the grace to continue what she was doing and grant me some privacy. I could feel the panic rising, spreading its roots in the pit of my stomach. A heavy stone ground its way around my guts, and my abdominal muscles screamed and squeezed. Would I shit myself right there in the middle of the cello section?

Inhale. Exhale. My eyes were unfocused, but Pam's blond head remained centered above my music stand. She was still playing; the music was continuing without me. The amount of energy she was committing to performing in this rehearsal was inspiring. I could do this. A little panic attack was nothing compared to trying to play G-flat scales at the breakneck speeds Brahms had marked in the music. I reminded myself, "It's ok to feel whatever this is. It's normal. Look at Judy."

With her hot-pink dyed hair, Judy stood out from the brown, black, blond, and grey heads of the orchestra. A little over a decade ago, she was diagnosed with breast cancer and had a double mastectomy. She is so healthy now that it is inconceivable that she ever had cancer at all. She often dyes her hair funky colors and has an easy and direct way of interacting with people that I never quite understood before my diagnosis. Only when she found out about my diagnosis did she talk openly to me about having had cancer.

Now, here she was, easily playing the music, her cancer a distant memory and a constant cloud all at once. She was doing ok; I could be ok, too. Her eyes flashed away from her music, her gaze meeting mine. She saw. She knew what was happening. I am never alone.

My heart was pounding so loud in my ears it was drowning out the sound of an entire orchestra. I was suffocating. I closed my eyes. *You can leave during the break,* I bargained with myself. *This was good enough.* I had accomplished what I set out to do: attend rehearsals. But if I quit after just two rehearsals and skipped out on the concert, I would feel I had let down everyone in our cello section. On the other hand, I had promised myself during cancer that I should not mistake my presence in this world as requisite. Here was an opportunity to put this theory into practice—I would not overestimate my importance in this orchestra. If I needed to walk out, would I have the courage to do it when all eyes suddenly fell on me?

Inhale. Exhale. There would be no hiding my weakness and fear. Judy already knew I was struggling, and my stand partner had seen me stop playing. Surely Pam could hear that no sound was coming from the person directly behind her—she would understand. I had all the time in the world to let this feeling pass. No one was judging me. In fact, it surprised most people I was at the rehearsal in the first place. That had to count for something.

While concentrating on playing my part, I forget just how vibrant and visceral the vibrations from all the instruments of the orchestra are. Even though my cello was silent now, I could feel it between my knees and against my chest, resonating in sympathy with the orchestra. I closed my eyes and allowed myself to sink into those vibrations. The sound of the orchestra was overwhelming, my ears screaming for silence. After the quiet solitude of all the months I spent cloistered at home, would it surprise anyone that the volume of an orchestra would overwhelm my delicate systems and leave me feeling weak and overloaded?

My body was shaking, nausea was rising in my throat, but I was still breathing. "You're ok," I whispered to myself. I ran my hand along the front of my cello feeling the tiny grits of rosin that had flaked off my bow, clinging to the wood. "It's a heavy burden being a young cancer survivor," Jeremy's words echoed in my head. And right at this moment, I was feeling the full force of that existential burden crushing my trachea. *Inhale. Exhale.*

I listened to the music swirling around me, letting it guide my thoughts back from the panicky edge I was teetering on. Now I understood Ella's exasperation when she described the well-meaning inquiries of her coworkers. She had said, "I hate it when people come up and ask, 'How are you doing?' No matter how I answer them, they tip their head and go on to say, 'How are you *really* doing?' As if they are in on a joke that I'm not doing well."

This had already started to happen to me. People were making me feel as if I were living some sort of lie, deluding myself into believing that my obvious good health was not to be trusted. Already, people were looking for a deeper answer—a hint that I was still suffering or hiding bad news. Or worse, like they wanted me to know they knew things were not ok and were offering me a tacit invitation to confirm their insider information.

Thankfully, I only had to live in this panic for a few minutes—Chuck announced a 10-minute break as soon as he stopped the music. I stayed in my seat while everyone else got up to stretch their legs. Judy made her way through the music stands, stepping over instrument cases strewn on the floor between the chairs. Once she reached me, though, she did not reach out and try to hug me. She sat in the empty seat next to me and placed her hand softly on my knee. She was treating me the way I treated Dusty when he was afraid, not grabbing and cloying, but instead helping me create a safe and secret cave in which to hide out for a few minutes.

"Are you sick of people asking how you're doing?" Her voice was soft, but her eyes were piercing. I knew she could see what was really going on. "People still ask me how I'm doing, even after all this time," she sighed.

I told her I was experiencing a panic attack and how she had nailed the cause. "Just when I've gone a few minutes without thinking about cancer, someone brings it up. Why do I always have to tell everyone about my cancer?" I blinked back tears, and she smiled gently.

"They're curious, and concerned, but they don't understand that sometimes we need to forget about cancer," she continued, reaching for my hand and clasping it in hers.

"I'm just so tired of talking about it. I just want to play my cello in peace," I whispered. There were so many reasons I was having this panic attack right now. It would be impossible to list them all, but Judy inherently understood them all, even if I did not put names to them.

"I know," she squeezed my hand. We sat like this together while she helped me regain control over my breathing. I was relieved that other people left us alone; perhaps the cave was real.

She gave my hand one more squeeze and asked, "Is it finally hitting you that no one thought you'd still be here now?"

My inhale was reflexive, my eyes stung with tears, and I squeezed her hand back. "Yeah," I whispered. My throat was tight, and my legs were trembling.

She patted the top of my hand. "I know, sweetie. I'm not supposed to be here, either."

The break was over, and the rehearsal resumed. A different piece of music was swirling around me now. What started as chaos short-circuiting my brain was now music slowly coming back into focus—the familiar chords and melodies finding their way through the shaky panic and straight into my heart. *Inhale. Exhale.* My chest was loosening. Pam's head was again moving hypnotically to the music. Judy's eyes softened, and she flashed me a quick smile across the orchestra.

Inhale. Exhale. I turned the page in my music, picked up my bow, placed it on the string where it belonged, and pulled it slowly to produce a deep bass note that vibrated against my chest, welcoming me back from my detour. I was ok.

Inhale. Exhale.

Scanxiety

12:30 a.m. Ugh. This was a bad sign—this was going to be a long night. Historically, waking up an hour after I turn off the tv means I will be awake for most of the night. If this were a Las Vegas Sportsbook, I would put good money on me waking up again at 1:30 a.m., 2:45 a.m., 4:00 a.m., and 5:00 a.m. At which point, knowing my alarm was set for 5:45 a.m., I would just have to resign myself to lying there awake, waiting for it to go off.

I thought I had a good handle on my anxieties heading to bed tonight. My stomach was not full of butterflies, and I'd had a great appetite at dinner—in fact, I could have probably eaten another snack before bed since I was feeling some fresh hunger pangs while brushing my teeth. There had been no obvious signs of stress or worry all day. Maybe, just maybe, I would not be one of those cancer survivors who worried about every single scan. Perhaps I struggled in other areas, but I felt emotionally healthy—as far as the infamous *scanxiety* was concerned. Tomorrow was my first PET scan since my reversal surgery in September, and I felt an unscientific certainty that it would go well.

My little alien co-pilot had other plans. My scanxiety was going to manifest as confidence, hunger, and insomnia. Not the kind of insomnia with butterflies in my stomach or as electricity buzzing in my legs which forced me to get up and walk around the dark house. My head was not full of chaotic thoughts or focused on specific worries. It was the kind of insomnia that prevented me from getting some solid REM sleep, and the kind where my head was eerily silent every time I woke up.

It did not surprise me when my first prediction came true—the next time I awoke, my watch read 1:24 a.m. Pay-out number one. Louis was snoring softly next to me in the dark; Luna was in her bed on the floor below my side of the bed, snoring louder than Louis; and Dusty was...well, I had no idea where he had been spending his nights lately. He was probably taking advantage of us being asleep and camping out on the expensive sofa he was never allowed on during the day. My ribs ached, so I tried to get comfortable, thinking about how I wished he would come back to sleep with us in our room again. Maybe if I made as much noise as possible as I rolled over, Dusty would be curious enough to come check out what I was doing. I hoped he would lie down next to me so I could stroke his fur until it lulled me back to sleep.

Two days ago, I had taken the dogs for a hike—our first hike together in a while. Because the rains had kept us indoors for weeks, we were all going a bit stir crazy in this unusual weather. Every time I bumped the basket where I kept the dogs' hiking gear making the bear-bell jingle, the dogs would come running, forever hopeful. But I would not take them out while it was still muddy; I had no interest in wrangling them for baths the moment we got home.

A week of solid sunshine after the rains finally stopped meant I could take them out again. We would brave whatever mud and water was still hanging around. Happily prancing along the main trail, we encountered our first obstacle: a wide rushing stream, about 3 feet wide, crossing the turnoff to the Miranda trail. Carefully stepping on the large rocks that formed a natural steppingstone bridge, my feet stayed dry. The dogs dove right in and splashed across. It was too late now to worry about keeping them clean. Who was I to squash their fun?

"Let's go see *Miranda*!" I called to the excited dogs. Taking the turnoff onto the trail, the dogs' excitement spiked when they realized where we were going.

We had to jump across another narrow stream that had washed out a low part of the trail. The rushing water adding an element of excitement for the dogs, and a mild panic for me. Not exactly the most coordinated person these days, I was still learning to compensate for the neuropathy in my feet, which left me with numb toes. Balance was tricky. We made it across; Luna was tugging and enthusiastically pulling me up the narrow trail. Holding her back just a little, I followed behind, allowing myself to fully indulge in the simple pleasure of enjoying the warm sun with my dogs.

When I hike by myself, sometimes I get stuck inside my head and I forget to fully marvel at how amazing our world really is. It may hurt my legs to walk through the thistle patch, but when I am with the dogs, I hardly feel it. I get so caught up in their excitement about what might be around the next corner that I hardly feel the painful scratches.

The trail is a simple loop over and around a wild hill. The view from the top is worth the long climb. The first half of the loop is a sandy trail, climbing up in full view of the morning sun, while the second section is a rocky descent through boulders and tall scraggy desert manzanita trees. The temperature difference between the two sections of the trail always catches me off guard. Often, I take off my vest at the start of the loop, forgetting how chilled I will be on my way down. June Gloom was in full swing, which meant cool morning temperatures in the weak sunshine. The dogs were making me sweat, though.

The recent rains had washed out parts of this trail. Grapefruit sized rocks littered the path and might as well have been boulders coated in water and fresh mud. They made for an obstacle course, promising to twist my ankle at every step. It was no longer a joke—I really could break my ankle if something went wrong. I forced the dogs to keep my slower pace and chose my footfalls as carefully as I could. The trick is to step in the grass off the trail, avoiding the wet leaves and mossy rocks. Parts of the trail, though, are steep and narrow, winding between the rock wall on my right and a drop-off into the deep canyon on my left. The options to avoid the slippery spots were not always available.

Of course, with all this attention to caution, I was bound to fall. My feet slipped out from under me, and I crashed down square on my ass. My tailbone took the full force of the impact; I was convinced that I had broken something. Perfect. I survived cancer, was on my way to wellness, and now I would have to spend the next six months nursing a broken tailbone.

The dogs, surprised by my fall, stopped to check on me. Luna stood in front of me, her nose exploring my legs and shoes, presumably to see if I was still the same person she had begun this hike with. After giving me a thorough sniff-down, and satisfied that I had not transformed, she took up her position as the lookout. She faced away from me, standing perfectly still. Luna is the most professional dog, our fearless pack leader scanning the trail ahead for danger. Dusty and I have a much different relationship—he is at the bottom of our little pack. He walks behind us, the guard and expendable pack member who would give his life to protect me and Luna. He was now behind and above me, standing on the rock ledge that I had just slid off, his face level with my head. His nose pressing into my ear, he gave my earlobe a reassuring lick.

"Good boy," I said to him, leaning my head closer to him. He stood patiently at my shoulder, watching me carefully. I stayed down, doing a quick self-assessment of the places I was feeling pain. My tailbone smarted from the initial fall, but overall, I felt alright. "I'll probably have a bruise on my ass," I told Luna when she looked back to see why I was still sitting there and not moving.

There was a strange, seemingly unrelated pain in the center of my chest. *Great. And now I'm having a heart attack.* I concluded I probably moved my arm wrong as I tried to catch myself in the fall. After a few minutes, I picked myself up, and we finished the hike. It was too wet, too muddy, and too treacherous to attempt any extra trails with my shaking legs. The whole thing had left me rattled. Besides, I had decided to put off breakfast until after the hike. Therefore, my hunger, and not the fall, was the official excuse to head home early. Luna, for as much as she loves to hike, always believes we are going home when we reach a particular spot in the park. Usually, I try to avoid that intersection of trails until I want to leave. Today, I would use her bad habit to my advantage and take them straight to it. Luna got the hint and led us the rest of the way back to the Subaru parked on the street at the entrance gate.

When I got home, I told Louis what happened. He could see that I was freaked out by my fall. "I'm turning into an old lady!" I moaned.

"Nah," he laughed. "You just proved chemo doesn't cure klutzy."

This fall was the main reason I was having trouble sleeping two nights later. The discomfort in my chest had grown into an obvious pain. Anytime I tried to raise my arms to shoulder height, the center of my chest screamed in agony. I learned through a quick internet search that the sternum often absorbs the energy of those kinds of direct impacts on the tailbone. I would be ok, but it would take time to recover. I took two Advil before bed, hoping this would help, but it barely touched the pain.

Not only was I having difficulty getting comfortable, but when I fell asleep, the slightest movement caused the pain to return, waking me up. At 4:00 a.m. (I was on a roll with my winnings) I was up again. This time, Louis was already awake.

"There's a skunk outside the window," he said. He hardly needed to tell me. Though all the windows in the house were closed, the smell was overwhelming. The dogs were awake, pacing in the hallway. A skunk had sprayed them a few weeks earlier; we all knew how horrible that smell was when it got into their fur, and this was definitely bringing up memories.

"Do did you hear a fight or anything?" I asked.

Louis crawled out of the covers, kneeling on his pillow so he could look out the window above our headboard. "No," he said as he got back under the covers. "I'll bet a coyote got one."

We pulled the quilt up just enough to block our noses and made jokes about a reverse Dutch oven. "I'll check the security cameras in the morning and see if we can hear anything," I decided. The camera set up in the back of the house usually catches every animal sound for miles, so even if the skunk or his attacker did not appear on screen, we might still hear what happened.

We could not get back to sleep. The acrid skunk spray burned our eyes and noses, and we were all riled up in the excitement, laughing and chatting. I was losing hope that I would get enough sleep. During my previous PET scan in August, I fell asleep inside of the machine—I was still weak and reeling from the difficult radiation treatments. I supposed I could nap in the machine today if I had to.

At some point I dozed off, avoiding the 5:00 a.m. prediction, sleeping all the way to 5:40—five solid minutes before my alarm would go off. *Not bad,* I congratulated myself. Alarms always scare me; at least I would avoid that jolt of adrenaline. Louis was already awake, so I shut off the alarm. He got up and went to the kitchen to make his coffee, while I slid out of bed and into the shower. My chest was killing me, so I stood under the hot water a little longer than I normally would, which helped. Because of the 6-hour fast before the scan, I could not take another Advil; I would have to tolerate the pain until I got home. After all that I had been through this year, I could survive a few more hours of discomfort.

"I guess I was nervous about the scan after all," I finally conceded. We entered the Disney Family Cancer Center and made our way through the back of the lobby to the familiar waiting room of the radiation department. "I thought I wasn't nervous. I was feeling good about this one."

Louis put his arm around my shoulder as I filled out the patient questionnaire. "Well, sometimes anxiety doesn't feel like anxiety. I think falling on the trail and not being able to sleep last night are pretty good symptoms." He gave me a warm squeeze. "It'll be ok. You'll see."

My greatest source of strength and encouragement, Louis has a way of deeply understanding me. I leaned my head against his shoulder, taking a break from recounting my extensive surgical history on the form.

I did not want to cry in the waiting room in front of the other patients. When I was bald, I felt entitled to burst into tears wherever and whenever I pleased. Everyone could plainly see *she's got cancer* and cut me some slack. My hair was now long enough to look like a regular short haircut. I no longer had the luxury of counting on the sympathetic smiles from strangers, so I blinked back the tears.

A few minutes later, the nurse led me to the room with the radiation symbol on the door, where I was first given a blood glucose test. Next came the syringe encased in lead that injects the radioactive tracer (F-18, Fludeoxyglucose). Again, I was thankful for my decision to give up eating added and processed sugar. Here was another injection which contained glucose meant to bait the cancer into consuming the important stuff—in this case, the radioactive tracer. Any cancer cells in my body (in fact, any cells with abnormal activity) would greedily metabolize this substance and "light up" on the PET-CT scan images. They use this as part of the process to diagnose many types of cancer; it is certainly how they tried to diagnose my cancer a year and a half ago. I wondered if there were any rogue cancer cells in my body, starved for sugar, munching on their specially prepared sweet nuclear treat.

While sitting in the room for the required 45 minutes uptake period before the scan, I received encouraging texts from Suzy, Lori, and Vicky. Alice had texted me earlier that morning to tell me that worrying would not change the outcome of the scan—if I could make peace with that, then I could face whatever the results showed.

Despite the nagging pain of my tailbone against the hard scan table and the dull ache in my chest while holding my arms over my head, I still dozed off a few times inside the machine. When the scan was over, the technician told me they would post the results to my portal in 2-3 hours, and then my oncologist would call me. I knew that Dr. Jacobs' day usually began at 5 a.m. with his rounds at the hospital across the street, which meant that he routinely ended his office hours around 2 p.m. Sometimes one of the nurses would call after Dr. Jacobs left for the day, but it was unlikely I would get a call that afternoon. I planned to spend the afternoon watching for the notification that the results had been uploaded to my medical portal.

As predicted, my phone let me know that something was happening. I clicked the link, logged into the app, and stared at the newest test result posted to my account: "Study Result, PET-CT Scan." I opened the document. Not surprisingly, the Head/Neck, Chest, and Skeletal scans were normal. I was relieved that the scan did not show a broken tailbone from my fall.

The only section I care to read is always listed last. The moment had come. How successful were the chemotherapy, radiation, four surgeries, and six months of adjuvant chemo?

Abdomen and pelvis:

Normal physiologic activity within the kidneys, ureters, bladder, and gut.

No mesenteric or presacral PET avid adenopathy within the pelvis.

No hypermetabolic asymmetry to indicate neoplasm on this current study.

IMPRESSION:

Negative PET-CT fusion scan

No abnormal neoplastic activity

Stable appearances over time

I printed the results right away and carried them across the hall into Louis' recording studio. He and a colleague were working on a project together, but they were more than just work buddies. These two were friends, even if Louis (so much like me) had been hesitant to build that friendship all those years ago. Michael and his wife had seen me a week before my cancer diagnosis the previous December, both wildly concerned by the way I looked. Through everything, Michael kept track of Louis, never letting him go through his part of this alone. So, it seemed fitting that this friend, who had been there for Louis during the scariest moments, would be witness to the breaking of some good news for once.

I normally wait to hear a pause in the music before I open the door, especially when Louis is in the studio with someone else. But this time, I burst through the door, Louis cut the music, and I handed him the printout. He read it quietly at his workstation. I could see his eyes roving over the paper. I imagined he had the same issues with literacy that I did when reading these scan results. He read through the scan several times in silence before he looked up at me. "This is amazing," he said finally, standing up and pulling me in for a hug.

Michael got up from his seat and moved toward the back of the studio. "I can go outside and give you a minute," he offered.

"No, no!" I laughed. "This is all good stuff!" For once, Louis had a friend who could focus on him during a happy moment. It was his turn to experience the importance of having a team behind him. I was glad when I walked back across the hall to my yoga-slash-music room to hear the two of them talking about this crazy year we had all just been through. Their muffled voices carried through the door, peppered with laughter and happy talk.

There is a lot to celebrate. But I was not sure I could trust the scan. I was still calling myself *technically* disease free, but this scan made it look like my body *was* disease free. These were words I would not say out loud. *No visible signs of disease* continued to feel like the best description. I had made it through one more scan, in a long life of scans. Although there was no telling what future scans might reveal, this one was unremarkable. And this one was the only one that mattered.

Ever so quietly, a little voice near my ear whispered: *Today, you're disease free.*

Part 4

"It's a heavy burden being a young cancer survivor."
–Jeremy Reynolds

Sun Spots

When I think of my college friends, I am at a loss as to the best way to describe them and our four years together in music school. Vignettes flash through my brain that would mean nothing to anyone else besides us: the oboe reed making room, and making sacrifices at The Shrine of the Reed Goddess, which was just a pile of broken and rejected reeds tossed in the corner of the desk under a childish crayon drawing of a stick figure woman; James doing his *Superman* routine outside my practice room window; Jayne making me laugh so hard once I peed my pants; Saturday night parties in the dorms with people with nicknames like "Booter," "Jesus," and "Lucky"—Evan mixing unholy cocktails out of whatever illegal alcohol we all had hidden in our dorm rooms, an infamous concoction of his, which I dubbed *O'Kahuna*, (mix of Kahlua, Malibu, and Bailey's Irish Creme) should make it obvious how "Booter" got his name; walking through the snowy campus with Jeremy late at night to get a grilled cheese at the snack bar during practice breaks; wiffle ball on the quad on Sunday mornings and pinball after lunch; the sound of a plate shattering after we dropped it down the dorm stairwell just to see what would happen; New Year's Eve when we drove up to campus to watch the lit up tower dorm windows change from '95 to '96. I remember a lot of laughter, a lot of holding hands, and boundless joy. Somewhere in all that fun, we went to classes and earned our degrees. My memories are less of academia and more of the laughter of my friends.

How can I ever truly capture the essence of those friends with mere words? Nothing short of impossible. The bonds we made were outrageously close. Graduation did not change the nature of the friendships. It might be a little more difficult to see each other as often as we would like. But these bonds are for life—no matter the miles, no matter the time, with just one text, phone call, or email, those friends are right there beside you once again. It is impossible to explain these relationships, so it is much more productive just to say these bonds exist and know the context is universal.

When I announced my diagnosis, one of the very first people to contact me privately was Jeremy. We last saw each other in person in 2019, just after he had finished treatments for non-Hodgkin's lymphoma. We passed the afternoon in a coffee shop in downtown Los Angeles, trying to catch up on the previous ten years. That day, I did not grasp the severity of what he had been through. He made it clear that he had gone through his treatments in private, and it was not something he really cared to talk about. Now that I have been through cancer myself, I completely understand his decision—I, too, have little interest in repeatedly recounting my story every time I visit with someone.

Could I have supported him properly if I had known what was happening when it was happening? If I am to be honest, I sincerely doubt it. I was still blessed with a lingering form of innocence. I never really understood what cancer meant for people my age. The only direct experience I had with cancer involved grandparents and the older parents of my friends. I did not know anyone my age who had cancer, much less a close friend like him. I would have been utterly useless; I doubt I could have been there for him in the right way.

Jeremy was a voice in the dark throughout all my treatments. He never hovered, never injected himself into my experience, and he never waited for me to reach out to him. He checked in at all the right moments, called me when he knew texts would not cut it, and whether he realized it, he was integral to keeping my spirits high. He was the one that told me as long I was laughing more than I was crying, then everything would be ok.

Despite the clear scans piling up on my desktop, the very real symptoms of PTSD continued to flourish and grow. I can type and type about the different ways it affected certain aspects of my post-cancer existence, but the fact was that it infiltrated every single part of my life. I tried to quantify it—how it affected my ability to get back to work, or my relationships with certain people, or my appetite, or energy levels. It has no regard for where I am, how great my day is going, or how long it has been since my last panic attack. It only cares to remind me it exists. When I have gone several days without an episode, when I seem to be getting comfortable again, it pops in to say hello.

Panic attacks rear their ugly heads at the most surprising moments. For several weeks, they had become an almost nightly occurrence—striking out of nowhere while we were watching tv in bed. I was reaching a point where they were so routine that I was ready for them when they happened. It was the ones that struck during the day that scared me the most.

There was no rhyme or reason to what might set me off. Was it a sound? If the door squeaked a certain way, it would remind me of the 5-FU pump, and bring on a wave of nausea. Ella told me stories of vomiting at work when the fax machine would kick on, making a sound too much like her chemo pump's servos. At night, when everything is quiet, I can still hear the sounds of my chemo pump. I wondered if my brain would ever let me forget it.

Sometimes, a smell or a flavor would hit me the wrong way. One day I was avoiding a particular food only to be struck by a craving for it the next morning. I learned that just because something caused a reaction once, it did not mean the same thing would do it again in the future. I was flailing and struggling one morning while Louis and I were watching tv—I had an unexpected reaction to a sound in the show. I struggled to come down from that scare; but I did it. My husband supported me through it, and afterward we talked again about the importance of therapy. I was still resistant to seeking professional help. The panic attacks were as real as my stubbornness. Why was I hesitating?

Later that afternoon, Jeremy called to check on me; we mostly shared about our post-cancer recoveries and reassimilation into our previous lives. After I told him about the panic attack I had earlier that morning, he immediately gave me a brilliant piece of advice: *face down the hard emotions now*. It will be so much more difficult if I ignore these problems now and expect to face them in the future. By then, I may not be as well equipped to recognize the root cause. Grief does not always present with obvious symptoms years after the initial event.

It seemed so obvious, but he had named what I was feeling: grief.

It's a heavy burden being a young cancer survivor.

This was all I could think about now. Grief was officially added to the growing list. PTSD was gorging itself on an ever expanding menu of triggers—it never refused to accept new menu items.

We talked for over an hour. Toward the end of the call, we managed to fit in a little laughing. A wave of sadness washed over me after we hung up. Jeremy and I were so rambunctious, carefree, and joyful in our youth. Our professors tried to seat us far apart from each other in class, knowing if we sat next to each other, there would be a constant low din of giggles and whispers, if not outright disruptions. We egged each other on like the guys from *Jackass* and laughed ourselves hoarse when we were supposed to be practicing late at night. Once, we took a sugar and caffeine fueled overnight road trip, stopping at every midnight diner between Columbus, Ohio and Ithaca, New York to order coffee milk shakes. We were drinking buddies, the best of friends, and musical soulmates. We were as close as friends could be, intensely fond of each other, and riotously alive when we were together.

We both had been struck with cancer. I could hear the effects in his voice. He is not quite the same carefree person he used to be. His wisdom comes at a high cost. I rage at something having been taken from the two of us. Flashes of laughter and joyful youth streak before my eyes. We can never have that back. Cancer stole lightness and freedom from the two of us, leaving empty chunks. Sometimes I am shocked at the sound of my laughter—what can possibly be funny anymore? Cancer canceled that piece of us. We are twin suns, each with a dark spot on us; we will never shine quite the same way again.

And that is so fucking unfair I can barely breathe.

Cleaving

Cancer survivors, patients in treatment, and those with no cure or remission can be burdened by grief, anxiety, and anger. Every single day since I awoke to my diagnosis in 2021, I have felt the effects of cancer on my emotional state. These days, I suffered from a straightforward fear about what the future holds, and swirling suspicions about what might be going on inside my body again as my CEA crept closer to 5 ng/mL. I questioned my supposed clean bill of health, knowing full well if cancer could grow out of control that one time, then obviously it can do it again. There is an overwhelming sadness about how my life has been profoundly changed without my consent.

I have been trying desperately to balance getting out of the house, out of my self-imposed quarantine, and back into my previous life. My first concert was fast approaching on the calendar, and I was feeling good about how I had handled the most recent rehearsal. It appeared as if I had been able to figure out how to avoid the public panic attacks and just enjoy being back with the orchestra. I felt entitled to pat myself on the back for a job well done. Considering the road I traveled to get to this point, this was quite the accomplishment—I had every reason to be proud of myself.

There was no question I had the courage to do these things; I just lacked the passion behind why I thought they were important in the first place. I count only eighteen months from diagnosis until this moment when I type these words. If a baby were born on the day I received my diagnosis, today it would be running around the house, bumping its head on the coffee table, and throwing my Tupperware all over the kitchen floor. It seems my cancer-toddler enjoys drumming on my pots and pans with metal spoons, hellbent on clanging my head into a jumbled mess. I cannot think straight for all the racket.

A big part of my post-cancer mental state involves mourning my first death, dealing with powerful grief, and having to face my uncertain future. Growing old is not guaranteed. Tomorrow, next month, or next year, may be as old as I ever get. This consumes my thoughts. I feel alone as I shoulder the crushing burden of fate.

I need time and space in which to mourn. Above all, I need to be allowed to mourn. No one should expect me to bounce back immediately or to act as if none of this mattered. This was the most traumatic experience of my life—sometimes I need sympathy. Sometimes I need to cry, and sometimes I need to be alone. No one needs to fix me just because I am introspective. It is not unexpected that I would be sad or angry, as well as jubilant or victorious. Sometimes I just need to talk about how I feel with no one jumping in to soothe me or cure me of those emotions. In fact, it is much better this way.

"I don't pretend to know how you feel," a friend said to me over the phone. "But I know what it feels like to need someone to listen to me." She has her own health issues to deal with. We have had plenty of conversations where we talk back and forth to each other, neither one offering solutions, just friendship and a sounding board.

Sometimes cancer survivors talk about themselves as who they were "Before Cancer" and who they are "After Cancer." I do the same, because it makes it easier to understand which part of my life I am referring to. My life does not follow a straight line from diagnosis to an uncertain future. I feel more complex and more beautiful than just lines and dots marking important events at various checkpoints. I feel less mathematical, less human, and more...organic.

Everything that came before my diagnosis feels like a dream I had about someone else. Those years were like the roots of a giant tree that had not yet erupted from the surface. The vast system of roots winding their way through the dark earth, searching for sustenance, meaning, and importance; always believing that something greater was just above the surface of the soil, if only I could erupt and feel the sun on my face. Awakening to my diagnosis was poetic—anesthesia induces our minds into a state completely devoid of time or consciousness. I went to sleep as the roots and awakened as a sprout.

Suddenly, I was thrust into the bright light and shocking pain that comes with being *awake*. I was like a baby at birth who is handed from obstetrician to nurse, placed on the incubation table, and fussed over to make sure they are stable. Oxygen is given, soothing words are spoken, and blankets are piled on top of us. The primal instinct to grasp anything that touched my hand was strong. The nurse had petted my hand to soothe me, and I grabbed on with the reflexes of an infant. Amidst the flurry of activity and cool masked nurses, one kind face came into focus—my husband—to welcome me with love and warmth. His dark brown eyes, shining with tears of love, fear, and relief, pierced through my protective newborn shield.

"You looked so young," Louis told me from my bedside. I made him recount the events of the surgery multiple times while I recovered in the hospital. I craved every detail of what happened to me from the moment I went under the knife until my memory returned twelve hours later. "The creases between your eyes were all smoothed out. You stopped carrying the weight of the world on your forehead." Since we met, he often presses a finger against the deep creases between my eyebrows, products of a lifetime of worry, trying to get me to relax my face.

This time, when I reached up and felt my brow, I could not feel the lines.

It was painful to be a little sprout breaking through the surface of the soil. It was overwhelming to feel the glaring sun on my face for the first time, and to know I had so much further to grow. These eighteen months flew by. This sapling grew quite a bit thanks to the right amount of sunlight, water, and positive energy. I have grown. I have changed. I have become someone new. The tough roots are still there—every one of them. Now, there is a line between them and the sturdy little sapling reaching into the sky with its new branches and delicate green leaves. Just like every other tree in a forest, I had to chew and claw my way to the surface, and then the real battle began as I learned I still had to struggle to reach for the sunlight.

There is no question: I am growing.

I am not sure why, but this makes me a little sad. Am I mourning that a lesser version of myself is no more? Am I frightened, knowing that growth is inevitable? Are there things about my old self I want to get back? Did I enjoy living in the damp, cold earth, as wayward roots reaching for nothing in the dark? Or am I sad because cancer forced me to erupt before I thought I was ready? Is it even sadness I feel?

Whatever it is, I need to honor that person I was before. The wide-reaching root system will always be deep under the ground beneath this new little tree—every branch that grows up toward the sky is the twin of a gnarly root in the dirt. Together they are life. Perhaps my lingering sadness comes from an implied expectation that I am supposed to leave behind who I was, cheerfully become a new person with indifference—just forget the roots below.

Instead, I should embrace the roots, the trunk, and the branches, making me whole and new. And it's ok to cry sometimes because healing and growing is extremely painful.

Coyote Walk with Me

Getting the dogs ready for a hike is like getting excited kindergarteners ready for school. First, we pack everything we need in our backpacks—Dusty carries extra water, some snacks, and a roll of poop bags; Luna carries the first aid kit, a small pair of binoculars, and wet wipes. In my backpack I have a large bottle of water, the dogs' collapsible bowl, my ID, phone, and trekking poles. Because I am ultimately a woman hiking alone in the wilderness, I also carry an air horn, a small thing of pepper spray, a bag of marbles (to toss at rattlesnakes sunning themselves on the path), a rape whistle, and a pocketknife. The world is an inherently predatory place; it would be negligent to pretend otherwise.

The dogs love to get into their backpacks, which makes things a lot easier for me. Luna whines, knowing what is about to happen, and Dusty stands by the door, hardly able to contain his excitement. They love to hike and, given how untamed and untrained they were when we adopted them seven years ago, this is a monumental accomplishment for them. Hiking seems to erase all the problems we have with leash manners. Both dogs are much braver in the wilderness, and it is a wonderful bonding experience for us all.

They still struggle with walking on sidewalks and streets. They are deathly afraid of small children, people, and other dogs. Rather than torture them on the half-mile walk to the hiking trails, I just pile them in the backseat and drive them to the park. When we arrive at the gate, I clip their leashes on to my belt, and let them explore within an 8-foot radius. Besides coyotes, there are bobcats, rattlesnakes, and off-leash dogs we might encounter on the trails. Keeping my dogs safe is my number one priority. They are never off leash, and we never go to remote areas where we might get into trouble.

But on this morning, I figured the dogs might like to hike a different set of trails. So, we headed to the other side of the park to tackle a challenging trail that I only attempt a few times each year. The Stagecoach Trail, otherwise known as Devil's Slide, is the historic stagecoach road they named the park after. It is a steep, rocky, treacherous climb on foot. It's hard to imagine the Overland Stagecoach Company dragging actual stagecoaches, loaded with people and luggage, up the mountainside in the 1860s. The channels cut in the sandstone by the wagon wheels are still there today. The climb is arduous, but at the top of the steep ascent is an amazing reward—a most spectacular view of the entire San Fernando Valley and beyond. Looking east, we see all the way to Burbank, over 25 miles away. The dogs love climbing the rocks, which distracts me and makes the journey much easier. On the descent, I have to rein the dogs in, so they do not pull me down. But once they figure out my pace, they take the walk in stride.

Usually, we take the left fork at the bottom of the trail, leading to another trail overlooking the train tunnel. Eventually, the trail ends at the paved access road that forms the border of the north side of the park. The pavement and gentle rolling hills give us a chance to stretch our legs and jog the next half mile, then we turn into the park on a trail that leads back up into the wilderness.

Today, though, we are not jogging. We walk, enjoying the cool morning, and all the interesting things to sniff. Luna seems to be more alert than usual, her ears pricked, and tail held high, walking at the very end of her leash, which puts some pressure on my waist under the belt. Dusty remains at my side, keeping perfect pace with my every step, and not showing the same amount of anxiety as Luna. We walked along for about a quarter of a mile in this manner, and I relaxed into the pace, chattering along to the dogs.

Suddenly, Dusty leapt forward. Struggling at the end of his leash, he spun around a few times and tried to pull away. Of the two dogs, Dusty is the best behaved on his leash. This was not like him at all. "What happened?" I asked. I felt fur against my bare leg and looked down. In Dusty's place, a dog of roughly his same size and color trotted along beside me. "Well, hello!" I said to the newcomer. "Are you lost?"

The dog looked up and our eyes met. This was no dog. It was a coyote!

For just a few moments, we had been walking side-by-side in complete harmony. She and I were now aware of the position we had put ourselves in. The dogs and I had unwittingly stumbled past her hidden den of pups. This coyote had snuck up on Dusty, maybe even nipped his tail, which startled him into jumping. She had been trotting along beside me for a few yards as one of the pack. Our fun morning hike was officially canceled. Now, there was only one thing to do: the dogs and I had to get out of there and she was going to escort us as far from her pups as possible.

She stopped walking and stood to watch us put some distance between us. I stepped up the pace and my dogs were all too happy to oblige. Luna wanted nothing more than to leave— she was pulling so hard on the leash I was being dragged behind her. I must not let them break into a run—that would provoke the coyote's instinct to chase. Dusty, despite his physical interaction with the coyote, remained carefree as usual. He settled back into his prancing gait, curled tail held high, and a goofy look on his face. Sometimes he reminded me of a cartoon dog, and right now, his lack of fear was the only thing keeping me from panicking.

I looked back to see where the coyote was. She was trotting along behind us, about 20 yards back, stopping occasionally to make a sharp barking sound. I worried she was calling the rest of the pack to her aid. Later that evening, I would research coyote vocalizations on a website run by a naturalist who writes about the urban coyotes in San Francisco, and discover that those sounds were not aggressive, but fearful. Coyotes are afraid of dogs, and this one was simply telling us she was scared.

I was scared, too! But we kept walking steadily onward, the re-entry trail back into the park within sight. I decided we would not take our chances on more trails with a coyote following so closely—we would stay on the road and eventually exit on to the main street, thankfully only a five-minute walk back to where I had parked the car. The dogs were going to have to confront their fear of walking on the street if we were to leave the coyote behind.

My breathing was heavy, my heart was pounding, and there was so much adrenaline pumping through my body that every muscle was moving of its own accord. A voice in my head repeated, "Don't run. Don't run. Don't run." For the next quarter mile, Luna pulled me forward with her leash, Dusty pranced his way down the hill, and I continued to look over my shoulder to watch the coyote. She never got so close to us again, but she continued to make her strange chirruping bark. She succeeded in her mission to keep her pups safe.

When we arrived at the main road, I looked back to see what happened to the coyote. I had not heard her nails clicking on the pavement as we descended the last hill leading to the park gate. My heart swelled at the sight of her, not more than 15 feet away, sitting perfectly still at the top of the hill we had just hurried down. Glowing in the warm morning sun, she looked ethereal, a messenger from a dream, a perfect statue in the middle of the road. Her fur moved in the breeze, giving the effect of a shimmer, and I was mesmerized. A perfectly painted wild creature with thick strong ears pointed at us, her amber eyes connected with mine. She and I stayed like that, facing each other, for quite some time before I led the dogs to the park gate.

The excitement of the experience has stayed with me. That coyote had been walking next to me. Few have felt the flutter of coyote fur against their skin. She lives in my memory as wild and miraculous as she did that day.

Coyote is always with me.

Dust

Sunset in Ventura County is a beautiful time of a summer day. In July 2021, our orchestra gave its first concert since the lockdown began, the performance getting underway just as the sun set and the shadows crept across the grass. The shade enveloped the orchestra, providing welcome relief from the soaring daytime temperatures. My old concert wardrobe desperately needed refreshing. I decided to purchase two new black tops, a black cardigan, a pair of black pants, and new black shoes to celebrate my return to the stage. This concert only happened two years ago, yet it felt like a lifetime had passed.

Flash forward to tonight, in the summer of 2023. The lockdown restrictions had been lifted for quite some time. We could perform indoors, which meant the orchestra could bring a more traditional experience to both the audience and the musicians. The last time I performed with this orchestra, we were outdoors in the park. So, this was not only my first concert back to work since cancer, but also the first time since before the pandemic that I had sat on an actual stage.

Now came the tough decision: what to wear. In my closet, there was nearly two years' worth of dust collecting on the shoulders of what had once been new concert shirts. I spent a fair amount of time staring at the clothes, contemplating whether I would throw things in the washing machine. With little time to spare, I had to make do with a half-assed cleaning attempt. I shook out the cardigan and used a damp washcloth to wipe the dust off what used to be my new pair of black shoes. This all seemed to do the trick.

Back in the closet, I had a more important decision to make—which of the two pairs of identical black pants would I wear? I had purchased one after the pandemic, during my original shopping spree to accommodate my lockdown weight gain. The second pair was a size smaller—I needed to buy this pair when I was rapidly losing weight ahead of my diagnosis because the other pants did not fit anymore. It was painful to remember that time when weight was falling off of me and my clothing hung from my bones.

It was a tough decision, but tonight I had to wear the smaller pants. I had only put on two pounds since finishing radiation—in fact, I was barely hanging on to them, almost a year later. My ass was still flat—making a straight line from my lower back to my hamstrings—not filling out the seat of any pants that I wore. But my face was becoming rounder and smoother again. According to the nurses, health and healing are most obvious in the face. As a teenager, I used to resent my round cheeks. As an adult, I reluctantly learned to tolerate this facial feature. Given everything that occurred in the past year and a half, I was relieved to see those cheeks again. Having a hollow face was a little unnerving. The significance of my round cheeks was not lost on me.

Pulling on the pants, I had expected to fill them out. I hoped that two pounds would make a significant difference in the way my clothing fit. But no. In fact, the pants were looser than when I had originally bought them. It was hard to disguise my frustration when Louis came in to help me fasten the button on the back of my shirt.

"Don't worry," he said, while he worked the hook and eye clasp. His fingers lightly brushed the back of my neck. "You're the only one who sees these things." Hopefully, the cardigan was long enough to cover my flat butt, just in case anyone did notice.

Sighing, I reminded myself that soon enough, I would put on more weight. Then, I would be able to move up to the larger pants collecting dust on the hanger. And, because of my body image issues, I would probably resent moving up to the bigger size. It would not be long before I would be trying to lose a few pounds again. There was no winning with me.

Dressed, it was time to pack the car. My fancy cello was already in its case, the music organized in my folder, and a seat cushion packed in my shoulder bag. I never used to bring my own seat cushion to performances, but now it was essential. The lack of padding in my butt cheeks made it difficult to sit on the hard stage chairs for hours on end. I found my lightweight music stand and battery powered stand light, packed everything into the back of the Subaru, closed the hatch, and began the 20-minute drive west to Moorpark.

As the personnel contractor, it is my job to hire the musicians in the orchestra. Throughout my treatments last year, I actually did this job from home. It was something that made me feel useful, productive, and normal. Now, it felt good to get back on stage with my colleagues, who had already given four concerts in this theater. Despite all the emotional setbacks of the past few months, I was excited.

Built in the 1920s, the small, tired art déco auditorium was still charming. Even though the stage was cramped, our little orchestra fit, and so it was the perfect place for us to perform. A member of the cello section, I had a seat at the edge of the stage. Being front and center was one of the exciting things about playing the cello. I never suffered from stage fright, even as a child; I love being on stage. It felt good to be back.

"Did you see the program?" A harried trumpeter rushed across the stage while I was warming up. He was brandishing the program and pointing at the list of musicians.

"No?" I said. What was he so upset about? Had someone misspelled the name of the conductor? Did we leave off one of the pieces we were playing? I followed his finger down the column of names of the musicians playing First Violin, Second Violin, Viola, and Bass. "No cellos!" I exclaimed.

Although it was my section that was missing from the program, he seemed more upset than I was. "What are we going to do?" he asked.

I told him I would talk to our conductor and let him know about the oversight. There was nothing else we could do 60 minutes before the concert started.

"I'll just introduce the cello section," Chuck decided when I let him know about the mistake.

Pam was listening from her seat and shook her head. "Please don't! No one reads the program, anyway."

The three of us laughed. I agreed with Pam, hoping he would do no such thing. But, if I know Chuck (and I think I do), he *would* make a fuss. I took my seat at the back of the cello section and faded into the crowd of black clad musicians as the first audience members trickled into the seats below the stage.

At exactly 7 p.m. the house lights dimmed, the stage lights came up, and our concertmistress walked across the stage to applause from the orchestra. The oboist played the "A," the orchestra tuned, and Chuck emerged from stage right for his bow. He took his place on the podium; a hush came over the theater as he turned to face the orchestra. The musicians raised their instruments. A soft collective breath was taken as he lifted his baton, and the first haunting notes shimmered from the muted violins. Ten minutes later, the music ended, the audience applauded, and various soloists took their bows.

While the musicians shuffled their music around on their stands, putting up the next piece on the program, Chuck turned to address the audience. He welcomed them and thanked them all for attending the concert. He encouraged them to make donations to the orchestra, and to buy coffee mugs, t-shirts, and refreshments from the sales table in the lobby. "And we also have a big omission from our program: the cellos!"

This was as much as I had hoped for—he would simply say something about the cellos missing from the program, wave his hand in our direction, and then continue with the concert. As predicted, he did gesture toward our little cello section of five players. But then, he kept on speaking, and I knew what was coming.

"Since they're not in the program, I'd like to introduce each of them to applause." He began with Pam, our principal player. She stood, smiled out into the dim auditorium to accept the applause coming from the faceless audience and the shoe-shuffles of the orchestra behind her. Chuck repeated this process three more times, each musician standing and receiving their applause. Tonight, I sat at the back of the section, so I was the only player left to be announced. "Last but certainly not least: Lisa Febre."

It took longer than it used to for me to get to my feet. The act of standing up seemed to drag on for hours. My hips creaked at the sudden movement; my back protested the unexpected requirement to straighten. Even now, almost a year later, my joints still felt the effects of the radiation. Consumed with my thoughts about how my body was fighting the simple movement of standing up, I heard a sound breaking through my cloud. The orchestra was clapping louder than the audience, and one musician hollered, "Yay, Lisa!"

Surprised, I turned to face the orchestra instead of the audience. "Wooooo!" someone shouted from the sea of musicians.

My eyes welled with tears, and I tried not to cry. I forgot about the dust on my shoulders and how my pants did not fit right. I forgot there was a concert going on around me.

After my reversal surgery, I had stood on this same podium and said, "I love this orchestra. It's an incredible feeling to know that you all love me back."

They were applauding not because my name had been left off the program, but because I was alive. All 75 members of the orchestra rallied around me when my diagnosis was made public. They fed me, they fed my family, some drove me to appointments, some came to my house to visit. Every single person in this orchestra sprang to action while I fought for my life. They were the ones who deserved the cheers and applause. I just rode their wave of energy.

The lone person standing on the stage, I savored this moment. Looking at this group who saved my life, I felt a surge of affection warming my chest and solar plexus—the opposite of the panic attacks I had been dealing with. Love surrounded me.

Ta-Dah.

Screams in the Night

Summer was rounding the corner into autumn and with the change of season, I was expecting a corresponding change of heart. The cooler days brought a friendly sort of orange sunlight and with it came more opportunities for me to be outside with the dogs. It seemed reasonable to expect that some emotional healing would naturally happen. Being outdoors more might distract me from my growing anxiety. And maybe nature would work her magic and fix me.

The dogs' daily routines are all tied to the sun. At the crack of dawn, they jump onto our bed, determined to let us know it is time to start the day. They were training me to wake up with the sunrise and teaching me to listen to the subtle and natural rhythms of my body. "Hooray, hooray, a brand-new day!" I cheered with them, day after day, week after week, as I dragged myself through my morning chores. For at least the first hour of every day, I felt enthusiastic and excited about the possibilities. But this was where the synchronicity ended.

The problems arose once it was time for me to rinse out my coffee mug and decide what to do with the rest of my day. Yoga or hiking would fill up a morning. Once I was finished, I did not know what to do with myself until dinner. Sometimes I had editing work to do on the computer, throwing myself enthusiastically into my *to do* list. A fast burn, though, means a fast fizzle. My interest in what I was supposed to be doing would wane. Five minutes would go by before I realized I had been staring out the window at the trees instead of the computer screen. I would get back to work, but I would find any excuse to stand up and walk around the house. I was unfocused. My yoga-slash-music room was quickly becoming my daydreaming-slash-procrastination chamber.

Shortly after the concert, I decided I would devote more time to writing and editing than to music. Although I loved being a musician, the upcoming book launch and new opportunities with other authors demanded my full attention. I spent much of my time writing a presentation for an event for cancer survivors and medical professionals at which the hospital, Providence St. Joseph, had invited me to speak. There were moments when I was excited, but always followed by moments of fear. Feeling a lack of confidence while thinking about my future made me feel dull and sleepy. My brain would rather shut down than accept the possibility of success on my new path. It had been difficult to build my music career. I always felt there were a lot of roadblocks and screeching hard turns. By comparison, things were going smoothly with writing; I did not trust that it was real. The Universe must be playing a cruel trick on me. Was the mouse amazed at how easily it got the cheese? I was bracing for the sound of a spring being released and the snap signaling the end of this impossible new dream.

Abby, my infusion nurse, continued to question me about my mental health at each of my Avastin treatments. She would ask about my appetite, my sleeping patterns, and my general mood. "I'm doing great," I would tell her. "I'm eating well, I'm sleeping pretty normally, and I'm feeling good." By this point, I was driving alone to some of these appointments; Louis was not always there to hear me lying to the nurses.

Every three weeks I answered her questions, then went home. There, I could truly ignore what was actually happening to me. I was ignoring my cello—in fact, I had already decided not to play the next concert; I was skipping multiple days between yoga practice. The poor dogs were patiently waiting for me to get them into their backpacks for hikes that never happened. I stopped cooking interesting meals and poo-poohed going out to dinner with my husband.

Louis worried about my caloric intake—he always wanted me to eat more than I was in the mood for, and he was concerned that my appetite was inconsistent. Some days, I would eat anything that was not nailed down. And other days, I could hardly bring myself to eat something as bland as a bowl of rice. My weight fluctuated within a 3-pound range, but by now I figured out how to dress for my weigh-ins so that the nurses in Dr. Jacobs' office would not see any change. I would weigh myself before deciding what to wear to the appointment. Facing the office scale, if I lost weight, I would wear jeans and a heavier shirt. But if I gained, I would wear yoga pants and remove my shoes. According to their records, I was staying very consistent. Mission accomplished: I was hiding in plain sight.

Friends were calling me more often, asking to meet me for lunch, and I was letting their calls go to voice mail. I was spending more time with Traci, lunches that stretched into hours. Suzy had landed herself in the hospital ahead of her upcoming radiation treatments on the spinal tumor, and I spent a day in the room visiting with her. Vicky had called me one afternoon to tell me she'd had *The Talk* with Dr. Jacobs. In this horrible conversation, he told her that all the treatment options had been exhausted. My emotions were swinging wildly between riotously fun days with Traci where I could hardly breathe for laughing, and heartbreakingly serious visits with Suzy and Vicky where it was all I could do not to scream at the unfairness of it all.

At home, I was coming apart at the seams, struggling to hold myself together like a normal person—crying while I stirred soup on the stove and bursting out laughing for no reason while I was in the shower. Meanwhile, every night in bed, before falling asleep, my throat closed, and I thrashed in the blankets while

Louis tried to calm me using the mantra my therapist had given us. The panic attacks were getting worse, not better.

My head was filled with an echoing chorus of shrieks and screams over an accompaniment of laughter and celebration. It reminded me of the sound a pack of coyotes made when it killed a cat in our neighborhood—the incongruity of the two wildly opposite experiences of the predators and prey, was playing out in my cells. They, too, were screaming for help, and I was afraid to listen.   Although I experienced, proportionately speaking, more moments of joy and hope, sometimes the fear was so intense that it would erase their delicate memory. Would I ever feel joy again, or would I choke on my grief?

Fear was creeping in as my CEA was creeping up. When I saw the office phone number pop up on my caller ID—Dr. Jacobs' office only calls when there is something to be concerned about between appointments—just like with the rest of my friends, I contemplated letting it go to voice mail. "Dr. Jacobs wanted us to let you know that your CEA has gone up again this week," the nurse's voice said plainly through the phone. I had just returned from a trip to Houston, Texas, where I sold advance copies of *Round the Twist* at the UOAA Conference. I was still coasting on that high—I sold all the books I had brought with me, which was a big deal. Now I was plummeting back to earth like a deflated hot air balloon.

In the weeks that followed, we would watch my CEA fluctuate within a small margin—only elevated by 1.0 ng/mL— but it might as well have been 100 points for how deeply it affected my mental state. Waking in the middle of the night, I imagined all the things that were happening inside my body. Was cancer growing out of control again? It seemed impossible, given how healthy I appeared. The only way to get back to sleep was to remind myself that it was only one point and I was still under the acceptable threshold of 5 ng/mL. "We'll schedule your next PET-CT and get our answers," Dr. Jacobs said to me in

September. Always the cool pilot in the right seat, he relieved me of the duty to fly my plane for a while.

Round the Twist officially went up for sale, and I threw myself into promoting the book, sharing the links to Amazon and Barnes & Noble, flooding my social media with pictures and ads, and building a slick-looking website for myself. I submitted the book for professional reviews, awards, and recognition. After reading my book, people looked to me for comfort, information, and guidance, calling me things like a warrior and a badass. They would send emails praising my ability to talk about bright hope and the power of positive thinking. They told me I was an inspiration to so many, and they were certain I was doing good in this world.

All the while, I was hiding the medical issues currently going on with me. What would they think if they knew I was not actually cured? Despite being in a book, my story was far from a fairy tale. This was real life. And real life does not have tidy story arcs which predicably wrap up under a colorful dust jacket.

I was careful never to use terms like *remission* or NED (no evidence of disease) in my blog or when speaking to anyone. When people used the word *cured*, I corrected them quickly. "*Technically* I'm disease free. No one says 'cured' with metastatic cancer." I held on to this as long as I could, but the truth was that period of my life was coming to a screeching halt. And I was going to keep it secret for as long as I could.

I was failing at being the character I had created in the book. There was a lot of pressure to balance. I continued to present my public face to the world—the positive, healthy, and hopeful façade. I could pretend to be all those things, as long as I wore that mask. When I was home, I could be the private Lisa who would sit on the floor beside the washing machine and cry because the effort needed to transfer the wet laundry to the dryer was emotionally crippling.

I would never give a truthful answer to the people who asked me, "How are you *really* doing?" I would protect myself until the bitter end and lie straight to their faces without an ounce of guilt. The genuine fears, the ones that whisper sweet nothings in my ear about recurrent, metastatic magic cancer, were not for anyone else to know about. No one could know that I laid awake every night worried about my liver, or that I was afraid I would not make it to my 50th birthday next May. Did people really want to know that I was already mourning the thought that I may not live long enough to see my son get married or hold any grandchildren? Could anyone ever truly understand that although I'd had two clear PET-CT scans this year, I would never truly be out of the woods?

Of course, I still had hope that I would remain healthy, my rising CEA was just a fluke, and soon enough it would go back down where it belonged. My goal was to remain *technically* disease free for as long as possible. But as long as these panic attacks continued, I was convinced my good fortune had run out. The world didn't know that in private, I was a fraud, cowering under the blankets, hiding from the screams echoing in the night. "Ha ha, fooled you," the little voice taunted.

Safe

Google "Life after cancer" and the little information provided is vague, if not predictable. The American Cancer Society, in a 2000-word article on their webpage, addresses the complexity of the subject. It mentions feelings of sadness, anger, and fear; suggesting that the survivor stay positive, exercise often, find emotional support, and to lean on spiritual or religious foundations. The information is good, but with one paragraph devoted to each aspect, it is hard to get a firm grasp on how deep the waters run in real cancer survivors.

Most days, I just sat on the back patio, reading, or playing solitaire on my iPad. I craved the warmth of the sun, but after a few minutes, my skin would be screaming. The Xeloda came with a warning to limit sun exposure, and I quickly learned why. My nose was a darker shade than the rest of my face. I had to wear sunscreen. But sometimes I resented the need to do this, so I skipped that step of my daily routine. Lounging on the patio, I would watch the dogs lazily dozing in the dirt under the trees or sniffing through the garden and munching on the olives that had dropped from our tree. A family of crows had built a nest in the neighbor's towering tree, so I would throw orange slices into the grass for them to snack on. The Phoebe flycatchers would swoop down and snatch tiny insects from the grass while a cloud of hummingbirds fought over the buffet of feeders hanging from our patio rafters. Louis' studio has a set of French doors that opens to the patio, so the serenity of the yard was often accompanied by a incongruent action-scene underscore.

At the start of the summer, I interviewed with the Colorectal Cancer Alliance (CCA) to be a mentor in their Buddy Program—a support system for newly diagnosed colorectal cancer patients to find non-professional help. I was perfect for this role; I was looking forward to giving support to someone who needed some hope and a safe place to vent their fears. My confidence wavered the moment the Zoom meeting ended. Who was I to be giving advice? Just because I had come through this first leg of my cancer journey, what would make me think I have any meaningful support to offer? Was I tempting fate? What if my cancer came back, and I went from being a survivor back to a patient again? How would that help anyone? How long would it be before I abandoned my Buddy because I could no longer support them? What also worried me was how attached to this person I would become. I love hard. Would I be able to give them the support they needed, or would I base my interactions on emotion and lose sight of my role? I guess my solution was to double down—I agreed to pair up with two amazing women named Grace and Jeanette. We instantly hit it off, and immediately, I was thankful I had done this—these relationships were helping all of us.

The malaise that was part of my daily existence was both a comfort and a curse. I enjoyed the luxury of relaxing and doing nothing for long stretches; I could hit the yoga mat late in the morning; I could practice my cello with the window open all afternoon. Whatever I felt like doing, it was all done without time restrictions. I had no job to worry about. The book was finished, so there was no more busy work to occupy my time. Although my first concert had felt like a success, I already decided not to play the next one. Knowing I did not have to download, print, and practice the challenging music was a tremendous relief.

By mid-summer, the hummingbird outside my window had abandoned that nest. Several weeks had passed since I had seen her visit the branch. To make myself feel better about her absence, I pretended she was the one who had built the new nest in the orange tree outside my kitchen window. I watched as she pieced this nest together with the strands of Dusty's blond fur left behind in the grass when I brushed him a few days earlier. She was on a branch so close to the window that I could clearly see all the features of her tiny face and the brief flashes of her tongue as she lapped the morning air. I was looking forward to next spring when the hummingbird might use this nest to lay her eggs and raise her babies. It would be an incredible experience to see the babies grow and flourish right there in plain sight while I washed the dishes.

Overwhelming sadness crashed over me as a salty ocean wave: *who says I'll be around next spring to see any of that?*

Again, I was feeling separate from everyone around me, even Louis. With no energy to face anything, I moped around the house. Staring at the dinner pots and pans, knowing I had to wash them, I would sigh and drag myself through the motions. Folding laundry was a drudgery, and making the bed was a battle between smoothing out the blankets and crawling under them. This was no way to live.

Every day without a panic attack was a victory, yet I was coasting through my life. At the grocery store, the colors assaulted my eyes; out to dinner, the noise of the conversations around me overwhelmed me; on the Fourth of July, the fireworks cut me to the core, giving me a milder version of the drooling, quaking panic that the dogs experienced. It was time to admit the obvious: I was not in control.

It had been over two years since I felt genuinely good. I had been dealing with cancer and drug side effects for so long that I no longer remembered what it felt like to be normal. I might be on Xeloda and Avastin for the next few years. Or worse, I might have a recurrence and start treatments all over again. By my calculations, I had a long way to go before normal returned. This realization brought with it its own brand of sadness.

Adjuvant chemo was nothing like primary chemo, so it was important to keep things in perspective. Xeloda comes with a lot of side effects, most of which are very mild and hardly bother me. Dry skin was something I could live with; constipation, acid reflux, and nausea could be controlled with medication. And even the mouth sores were of such a low level I could deal with them and still have the energy to complain about my altered sense of taste.

However, I still panicked whenever something slightly out of the norm occurred. The first time the drug gave me constipation, my overreaction was epic; I almost lost my mind. My guts were not moving. Like a giant machine with seized gears, the entire system ground to a halt. There was no bubbling gas, gurgling noises, or urges to go. I had no appetite at all, no desire even to drink a protein shake. It felt like cramming food into a completely blocked pipe. My belly was taut and sore. I tried to keep my composure about it. Louis would eventually remind me that I could not keep things like this to myself. I felt differently. We just spent a year emptying bags of poo together; at some point I should have a little bathroom privacy again. It was time we regained some sense of mystery in our marriage.

I was panicking despite myself. And thankfully Louis was empathetic when I burst into tears in the kitchen while he was making his lunch. "Why are you crying?" He held me close and kissed my ear.

"What if it's..." The unresolved sentence hung between us. I could not bring myself to speak my heavy burden out loud.

He pulled me back to arm's length and wiped my wet cheeks. "I know you're worried because of your CEA. But, Dr. Jacobs isn't rushing you into treatment. So we can relax until he says otherwise, right?"

I nodded. "But it's the same way this all started before." We would not soon forget the horrific pain, swelling, and constipation, which had been the most serious symptoms of the festering colon cancer.

"You're healthy. This is just because you've been on Xeloda for almost a year. You'll feel better when you poop." He smiled, and I believed him. Just to be sure, I called the office. Dr. Jacobs reassured me that this was a side effect of the Xeloda, to take laxatives, and it will pass. Sure enough, later that evening, everything did. After two days of being backed up and then several hours on the toilet, I was exhausted. I passed out around 8:30 p.m., something Louis knows I never do, which is fall asleep early.

Many things reminded me of the time before my diagnosis: the backs of my legs being sore from sitting on the toilet so many times in a day; the way my bowel hurt every time I had to go; not being able to empty my bladder because of the full rectum pressing on it from behind; the lack of appetite, the shaking, and the uncertainty. Enough to make the tiny little alien inside me freak out at the controls. I knew my cancer survivor friends probably went through similar moments, but they rarely, if ever, talked about them. We were all groping around in the dark, convinced we were alone. We never saw the room was full of other groping people.

Last year, while receiving treatments, I used my blog to vent and navigate my emotions. Most people would comment with something supportive; some would tell me they had learned something important about what people go through when they have cancer; and cancer survivors told me they had gone through the same things. Validation in those forms did wonders for my head. But I had stopped writing on the blog. In fact, I had not officially updated the blog since my reversal surgery, which meant that almost a year had passed since someone could act interested in what I had to say.

I was officially anonymous again, enjoying the freedom to keep everything to myself. My Facebook posts could be about things other than cancer; I could post about the book. The tome I created during treatments was now a bittersweet accomplishment. Everyone praised my devotion to the project. Some were even congratulating me on "being cured," having no information other than the way I looked, or the end of the book, as the basis for this declaration. I was afraid these comments would jinx my good health and somehow end my year-long run with *no visible sign of disease.*

It felt like no one fully appreciated just how scary and impossible this cancer was to treat—did they really understand how serious a Stage-4C diagnosis was? What had happened to me was unique—more common was what was happening to my friends. Two years later, Suzy was still struggling to get ahead of her cancer, which had metastasized despite all the chemotherapy she had this year; Grace was told she would be in treatment for the rest of her life and had to accept the idea of living with drugs; Vicky's treatment options were exhausted, yet she would kick and scream with all her might until the end; Lori had a friend recently diagnosed with colon cancer who was struggling to find a medical team that would take her seriously; and, of course, Jenn's death. These were all reminders of what cancer actually looks like. It was possible that people thought I was exaggerating because they were unaware that my situation was unique. Mostly, I looked and acted like myself again; people were getting the wrong impression about the seriousness of metastatic cancer. To them, I appeared to be cured. Dr. Quilici had said, "You beat the odds," not because he was being hyperbolic; he was genuinely amazed that things had gone so well for me.

It was scary and lonely to live with the burden of waiting for the other shoe to drop. "I don't think I can take this news at face value," Suzy's words continued to play out in my head. Grappling with gratitude for my current well-being, I also faced the constant fear of cancer's reappearance. I had a choice between moving on or holding on. Would I devote my energy to getting on with my life? Or would I waste it by shouting into the wind in a pointless exercise to convince everyone that I really did almost die?

The blog could sleep. Freeing myself from that ball and chain allowed me to experience my recovery without having to perform for an audience. Probably people were thinking, "Phew! Glad she's finally shut up about her cancer," and were glad to have stopped getting the notices in their inboxes that I had posted another intense, emotional blog for them to grind through.

I decided not to tell anyone about my steadily rising CEA levels at the end of the summer. I was done inviting an audience for these things. Whatever the explanation for this rise, it was all too scary, and too private. I needed space in which to flip out. The rest of my life was going to be about fluctuating numbers. Now was as good a time as any to practice keeping my mind on the present, and not imagining horrible things waiting for me down the road.

I had more pressing concerns at the moment. Like that our insurance company just sent us a letter announcing they were pulling out of California and our coverage would end on December 31, 2023. I had doubts about their willingness to approve new care requests until then, especially since they had already rejected the osteoporosis drug injections three times since my diagnosis last January. If Dr. Jacobs added any new procedures or treatments to my growing list of claims, I doubted the insurance company would jump to cover them. I was still waiting for my Social Security Disability Benefits application to process, and the hope that I might actually qualify for Medicare soon.

Before any of this could happen, the first order of business was to shop for a new policy on the California healthcare exchange. The idea of shopping for new insurance felt overwhelming. At least, with the passage of the Affordable Care Act, insurance companies can no longer deny new policies to people like me because of a preexisting condition. And cancer is the mother of all preexisting conditions.

Night after night, the panic attacks continued to sneak up on me while we laid in bed watching tv. I was seeing a hypnotherapist regularly now. The sessions left me feeling empowered, centered, and confident. Louis and I were using the tools she gave me to work through the panic attacks.

"We have billions of cells in our bodies, each with their own memories of the experience of cancer. Some of them have moved past what happened, but others are still struggling. These attacks are the cries of your cells." When she said this to me, the macabre duet of the screaming cat and the celebrating coyotes flashed through my mind. My body was still afraid of cancer stalking in the dark, not convinced the danger had passed. Right now, I am ok. We are all ok. Not all my cells had received the message.

Each night, when a new panic attack would grip my throat and chest, I repeated the words she suggested: "I am safe." I found new comfort as I spoke the words out loud, and Louis whispered them back to me in the dark. My head and my heart slowed, my breathing deepened, and my chest released. This is the closest I have come to an emotional cure on this journey. I was feeling empowered—I was taking control over my inner well-being.

The trick was to believe the words I was saying to myself. Nothing is happening to me. I am in my bed. My husband is lying beside me. Down the hall, Andrew is in his room. The dogs are sleeping soundly in their beds. I am safe.

And for the first time, as I breathed calmly again, I heard powerful words spoken clearly from an invisible ally beside my bed: *you are a survivor.*

Painted Lady

The days kept up their unrelenting slow march toward the biggest and most important of all the cancer anniversaries—my one-year post-primary treatment survival. No matter what lay ahead, this was a miraculous milestone no one thought I would live to see.

Twenty-one months ago, when I was diagnosed with cancer, the idea that I might one day hear the words, "No visible sign of disease," was outrageous. It felt like cancer would consume the rest of my shortened life. Instead, the steady flow of time brought healing and courage. Every morning I awoke to discover I felt a little better, a little stronger, and a little braver than the day before. It was possible to believe there would be a time when cancer was just a memory. I was free to hope for some good news at the end of this journey. "No visible sign of disease," Dr. Quilici had said. He had given me permission to be innocent again.

To celebrate this big day, I hiked by myself. I had a lot to think about. It was important that I spend time contemplating and appreciating how I was doing at this very moment. My CEA was holding steady at the new higher number; Dr. Jacobs was subtly preparing me for a coming storm—the PET-CT was looming in the coming weeks, and we all expected it to reveal the cause. I would have my answers as to how I was really doing. Would there be more surgeries? Would there be a recurrence? Would I need more chemo? Today, as the sun made its daily transit across the morning sky, did it really matter? I was alive *right now*, experiencing *this* moment, with no need to worry about things that were out of my control.

Walking from our house to the park, my mind flashed through the memories of the past year like a slideshow. And again, in a testament to my innate positivity, all those memories were happy ones: hugging my friends at my first rehearsal, lunch dates with Ella, funny texts from Lori, the scent of Vicky's hair, Suzy's smile, and Dr. Jacobs' laughter when I presented him with the joke shirt I had made for him—a thumbs-up photo of me with the caption "I saved Lisa Febre's life and all I got was this lousy T-shirt." It had been a good year with so many reasons to celebrate.

Attacking the sandy, steady climb of the first half of the Miranda Loop forced me to focus on my breathing—it was getting shallower as I pushed myself unnecessarily hard up the hill. Why *was* I rushing up the hill? The dogs were not with me; this was not a race. I took a moment to stop in order to get control over my breath.

Turning slowly in place, not wanting to lose my balance on the steep trail, I looked out at the San Fernando Valley stretched out before me. To the north, rocky hills stood between me and the horizon, a wild and untamed wilderness defining the edge of one of the most thickly populated cities in the nation. There were trails in those hills, and now that I was feeling better, I planned to hike those again. Through the haze, I could just make out the buildings of Burbank to the east. The building that saved my life was somewhere over there. Just below the hill on which I stood was our house. It was impossible to see it through the thick old-growth trees of our neighborhood hiding the rooftops. Regardless of whether I could see it, it was down there—the first house Louis and I ever bought together; the house where I had fought for my life; the house where we planned to live out the rest of our lives. My heart swelled a little, thinking about the incredible things that had happened in the ordinary house hidden beneath those ancient trees.

The hillside sloped downward, making me a little dizzy. Turning back to face the rising trail laid out in front of me, I marveled at the steep grade I was tackling. I was only halfway up the hill. If I took my time, leaned into my trekking poles, and enjoyed the process, I would be at the top before I knew it. Just like with my treatments, there was nothing to be done about what comes next. There was only the acceptance of the place I was now, and knowing I would not be there forever. *This is all temporary,* indeed.

Slowly, I resumed my climb, carefully deciding where to place my unsteady feet. The neuropathy that had been plaguing me since I had FOLFIRINOX last year was in full swing today—the bottoms of my feet were prickly, and it felt like there were stones in my shoes—but it would not stop me from enjoying this hike. Reaching the top of this first climb, I experienced that wonderful moment of relief. Just when it feels like I cannot climb another step, the ground has leveled off and everything feels easy again. The release that follows is truly magnificent. I secretly congratulated myself on reaching this point, even though it was never in question. It's just that sometimes I enjoyed acting as if this were a noteworthy accomplishment.

Onward I hiked, up one more rise toward the peak of the next hill, using my poles to press the overgrown nettles and thistles out of my path. I had almost worn shorts this morning, but now, seeing how many of the spiky weeds had grown here since the spring rains, I was glad I had zipped the legs onto my hiking pants. Finally reaching the very top, the exertion of the climb steadily fading, I could hear my thoughts again. And those thoughts were quick to turn back toward a year ago, when my survival was not guaranteed. After chemo had killed most of the cancer, the radiation had threatened to finish me off. For months, I fought a festering resentment toward the radiation, the thing which ultimately saved my life.

The radiation dot tattoos had been the primary proxy for that resentment. These tiny tattoos, about the size of a freckle, are common with radiation treatments—we get them during the planning session so the technicians can align us perfectly within the radiation machine every time. Although I have nine much larger tattoos on my body, it does not make me feel any better when I catch a glimpse of these dots in the shower. I hated them and wanted them removed or covered up; I wanted to gouge them out of my skin. Sometimes I thought I would like to have tiny bumblebees or hummingbirds tattooed over them. But then I would think, *what if the cancer comes back and I have to have radiation again?* They might need to use those tattoos. I was getting myself into a sad loop. It was time to change that way of thinking. Since radiation had happened during June and July of last summer, I spent the corresponding weeks this summer trying to adopt a positive view of the tattoos. It appeared to be working. Eventually, I saw them through the lens of compassion, loving kindness, and even as marks of an accomplishment. Microscopic badges of honor.

A year had passed since my reversal surgery; for most of the year, my bloodwork held steady, which I hoped hinted at calm waters for the foreseeable future. Of course, as soon as I relax, something always pops up. A recent phone call from Dr. Jacobs' office had set me on edge again. "Dr. Jacobs wanted me to call you before you saw the bloodwork results in your portal," nurse Brian said. "Everything else looks good. But he doesn't want you to freak out: your CEA is elevated again." Who me? Freak out? "The upcoming PET scan will hopefully explain what's going on."

I had to stop obsessing about all the reasons my CEA might be steadily climbing now. It could climb for any number of harmless reasons, including inflammation somewhere in my body. But more likely, it was cancer. Instead of dwelling on it, I kept doing all the things I have been doing to keep my body healthy: exercising, eating right, taking a fistful of supplements every day, and keeping a positive attitude. There was no point in worrying. Besides, there was nothing to be done, anyway. Dr. Jacobs told me not to freak out, and I was devoted to following his every direction. Whatever this upcoming PET scan might show, I would face it just like I had faced everything else up to this point. By trusting Dr. Jacobs and Dr. Quilici, following their treatments and advice, I had lived a year longer than anyone expected. *A year!* I was not just surviving—I was thriving.

Just as with yoga, hiking was not the same for my body as it had been before cancer. The incisions from all my surgeries had healed, but they had formed into large, itchy keloid cysts, and even a year later were still red and angry. I could feel the irritated stoma scar rubbing against the waistband of my hiking pants. My ankles felt stiffer, my knees a little creakier, and my hips had a little less swivel to them. *This is what it will feel like to hike when I'm 70,* I thought to myself. And then I rolled my eyes at my audacity. Who says I get to be 70? It was an incredible accomplishment to be hiking right now. I had gratitude for this day, this sun, the birds above me, and the breath flowing through me. This is the only moment any of this will be exactly as it is. I am alive today—the only day I have to live.

No matter how much time passed, how much I healed, how hard I worked on my mental recovery, I still fought the little voice that yelled, "This is so unfair!" Thankfully, that voice was silent this morning. I imagined the little alien who liked to pipe this over the speakers from the cockpit inside me was distracted. Like me, it marveled at the beautiful day, the number of lizards scurrying across the path, and the fluffy tail that disappeared into the scrub up ahead. I stopped in my tracks, hoping for a hint of the hidden coyote, expecting to hear light footfalls or the sound of fur through desert grass. It was always a special moment to see a coyote out on the mountain, their bright ochre eyes following my movements, thick ears pricked with curiosity. I wish I had seen more than just the tail today. Maybe that was all I was supposed to see—my coyote spirit disappearing into the complicated wilderness, unbothered by the heavy heart coming up the trail.

I reached the top of the loop, the halfway point, without even realizing it. As I crested the hill, the wound from the construction came into view. The summer months had been kind to the land, helped along by the heavy rains this spring. Chaparral and weeds had finally taken hold on the injured earth. The path, which I had been faithfully pounding hoping to keep it clear, was visible through the plant-life. Carefully choosing my footfalls, I began the descent into the wounded acre, shaking my head at how long it had taken for Mother Nature to reclaim this land. But, also amazed at how well it had healed.

After walking 20 yards into the wound, I stopped and turned toward the rocks that had been blasted. The manzanitas were throwing up their first tender shoots. For the first time since the damage happened, a field of wildflowers was in bloom. "We're ok," I said aloud to the field. We might be a little battered and bruised, but we survived. *Miranda* and I will never be the same. The flowers may bloom above the surface, but below them, there are deep alligator scars which will never heal.

I thought of Vicky. A dark shadow of sadness for my friend passed over my heart. I reminded myself that the pain I felt at her loss was directly proportional to how deeply she had loved me. Not everyone gets to have a friend like this, and I was lucky that our lives crossed—no matter how short our time together.

"I'm going to miss you so much," she had said to me at our final goodbye. Her voice was as real inside my head as if she had been standing beside me. However long I live, I will never forget her. My lower lip turned down at the edges and I felt a wave of loss flooding my eyes.

As if sent to find me before the tears made it past my eyelashes, a little moth flew inches from my nose. Distracted from my heartache, I watched its carefree flight path through the field. Unable to resist the chase, I stepped into the wildflowers without a thought for hidden snakes or rocks, trailing the moth until it landed on a purple bloom. It relaxed its wings open and revealed that it was not a moth at all. It was a Painted Lady. I watched as it lazily opened and closed its wings—first showing its grey underwings, then opening to reveal the orange and black pattern hidden within; then back to grey again. I reached out, hoping the dainty butterfly might climb onto my finger, and I was not disappointed. It reached out with its front leg, felt solid footing, and took a few gentle steps onto my finger.

"Hello there," I said to it, holding it up so I could see all the details of its face. It continued to open and close its wings in its slow and thoughtful way. "I'm doing ok," I told it. Its little antennae wiggled in my direction. We contemplated each other for a long moment. Then, with a movement like a whisper, it took flight. I watched as it flitted amongst the field of flowers that had overtaken the scar on my beloved trail until it finally disappeared into the thick scrub.

Overwhelmed by the moment, I realized just how lucky I was. How lucky *we* were—*Miranda* and me. We had been attacked, poisoned, injured, blasted, scraped down to the bare dirt, our roots dredged to the surface, our hair sawed off, our skin flayed back, and our guts reattached. Yet here we were.

Miranda was growing wildflowers and nurturing butterflies. I was doing the same in my own way.

"I am going to live, too," I said to the living and breathing land. With a surge of positivity, I stepped back onto the path. The second half of the trail would pose new challenges as it wound its way down the rocky and steep side of the mountain. After an emotional year, I felt ready to face the long hike through the nettles and thistles.

Acknowledgements

To survive one year past diagnosis is a milestone to be proud of. Even with all the bumps and bruises along the way, this year has been an amazing ride. Thanks to the efforts of *The Team of Grownups*, I am alive and kicking. The fact that I can cry and complain and laugh and rejoice is a miracle all unto itself. My love and deepest gratitude to those doctors whose unbending and unblinking belief in the right path propelled me every step of the way: Dr. Edwin Jacobs, Dr. Phillipe Quilici, Dr. Paul Menzel, Dr. H. Lee Kagan, and Dr. Taaly Silberstein.

My husband, Louis Febre, spent another sleepless year with knots in his stomach, and yet still found a way to carry me when I stumbled. I wish "in sickness and in health" was not the most worn-out clause of our wedding vows, but we can't choose the things life hands us. Very few people have a partner as devoted, compassionate, and empathetic as you, and I will never take for granted your unwavering love.

My son, Andrew Jenkins, encouraged me to keep writing, to keep learning, and to keep putting one foot in front of the other. He went from child to cheerleader nearly overnight. There is so much to be proud of as he takes his first steps into adulthood, though I'll always see him, in my mind's eye, wearing his Thomas the Tank Engine backpack and riding his little bike to third grade.

Lori Stone, the years keep ticking by and yet here we are still passing notes all day long to make each other smile. It doesn't matter how many miles are between us, you have been with me every step of the way, never once wavering in your belief that I have so much more living to do. If there was any magic involved in my journey, it was because you made me believe it was real.

Suzy Lee, you may be the toughest woman on the planet—I've seen what you do to cancer, remind me never to get in a wrestling match with you! Your grace and courage are so admirable you make my heart ache. Never stop believing that you are going to live to a ripe old age.

Traci Asher, an inspiration to all who cross her path, and somehow, I was lucky enough to have a full-fledged friendship with you. Like a ninja, you have shown cancer who is boss, and every time it dares rear its ugly head anywhere near you, you've grabbed it by the throat and forced it to the ground. You live hard and love even harder, and I am incredibly lucky to be on the receiving end. 1cancerpatient.com

Vicky Claussen, you showed me what unconditional love looks and feels like. The last words you said to me were, "I am going to miss you so much." My heart will always have a hole where once you lived. I will never, *ever* stop missing you. To Gary, Damon, and Kymm—thank you for sharing her with me, and for welcoming me into your family.

Pamela de Almeida, Ella Davies, Alice Sherwin—with an Army of badass women like you behind me, I had no other choice than to stand up straight and face this year head on. You pushed me out of my comfortable bubble to show me that my life was waiting for me, while reminding me that there was always a safe place for me to retreat. Cancer sucks, but our friendships became even deeper thanks to it.

Jeremy Reynolds, seriously, can we ever have a conversation where you don't make me laugh so hard that tears stream down my face? You have brought nothing but joy to my life since we met three decades ago, and that has continued through these dark years. How many people can say they have a friend like that?

Grace Hensley and Jeannette Kim, my Colorectal Cancer Alliance "Buddies." The Universe works in mysterious ways. I underestimated just how important belonging to this program would be. You are no longer strangers who were "assigned" to me, or mere pen pals; you are my dearest friends and I can't imagine going through any of this experience without you.

Christina Buckner, sometimes you may not feel brave, you may not feel strong, you may not feel optimistic, but you are more amazing than you realize. In your own way, you have inspired me to dig deep, to find gratitude for the little things, and to really appreciate just how young we all are. There is a lot of living left to do, and so many people want you around for the long haul.

Thank you:

To the heart of Black Rose Writing, Reagan Rothe, for taking a chance on a new writer—this could have gone sideways real fast! This new family not only saw me through the writing and editing of this book, but also stood by me during all the ups and downs of having cancer. BRW has created an amazing community of authors who support and cheer each other on. Special thanks to those who have become more than just work buddies: Christy Burnett, Dave Buzan, Troy Hollan, Niamh McAnally, Karen E Osborne, Toni Runkle, and David Seaburn. Thank you to David King and Richard Gilmore for the beautiful covers on this book and *Round the Twist*.

To Yvonne de Sousa and Barbara Luker, who illuminated a new path for me to explore. You recognized something in me I wouldn't have seen myself; your encouragement and support has changed my life. You are my friends, and ones whose writing advice I respect without question. You both said "Just write it down," at various points in this journey, and this advice gave me the rare opportunity to actually meet myself on the page. I truly believe we were meant to cross paths. I can't imagine my life now without you.

To all the nurses at the Disney Family Cancer Center who draw blood with the gentlest touch, puncture my portacath with a steady hand, and give the kinds of hugs that can kill cancer.

Brian, Letty, Lucy, Lori, Debbie, Abby, Terry, Trish, Nancy, Diane, Tammy, Cindy, and all the others who I may not have mentioned by name.

To my amazing support team, Rémy Leigh Peters, Martha Inofuentes-Likins, and Andréa Mikolajczak-Novicki. Sometimes it feels like you are a Greek chorus following me to offer immediate support and advice, but most of the time, it feels like you are my friends.

To the Moorpark Symphony Orchestra, the Board of Directors, and Music Director Charles Fernandez. There is pure magic among this group of musicians, and my heart is always on the stage with you all, even when I can't be there. So many people jumped to action when I was first diagnosed, and that attention never once wavered, even during this past year when I was recovering and doing well. I am still blown away that you all love me back…

To my family and friends: Melissa Brunsting, Adrian Febre, Benjamin Febre, Roberto Febre, Alejandra Febre, Daniela Febre Domene, Lorraine & Dick Gilmore, Ana & Joel Guzman, Claudia Guzman, Carolina Guzman, Emily Shearing, Joanna & Larry Smolen, Melissa & Todd Smolen; Gail Amendt, Satsuki Crozier, Helena & Michael Gatt, Amy Hately, Rachel Leshaw, Beth Lano, Tara Buckman, Pamela Bruchwalski, Charles & Ingrid Olobri, Rosa Robledo, Randy Weinstein, Steve Burch, Sharon Cooper, Rhondda Dayton, Jennifer Deirmendjian, Vic Deirmendjian, Geri Freeland, Judy Garf, Toni Jones-Lee, David MacDonald, Roger & Barbara Mason, Sean Matthes, Lynn Olson, Barbara Poehls, Gary & Phyllis Rautenberg, Andy & Martha Siditsky, Gail and Jeff Smith, Nicole Wright, and Miriam Wu. Even if I forgot to mention you here, know that the smallest gestures never went unappreciated.

Photo Album

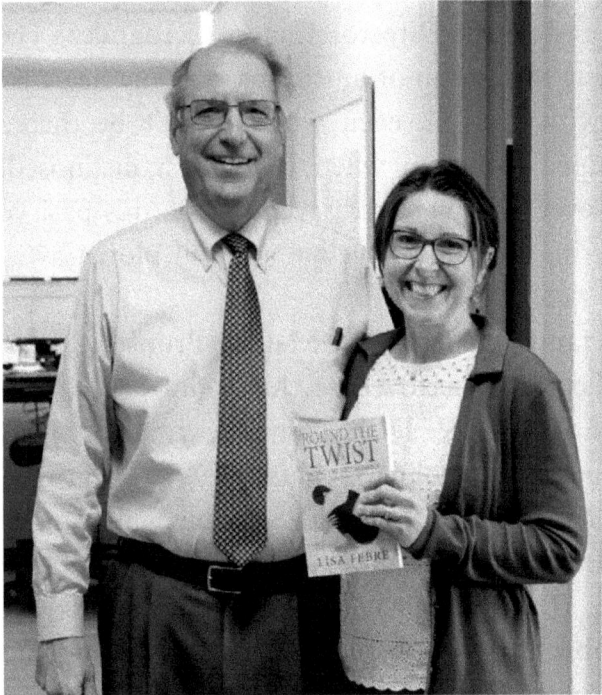

Dr. Jacobs

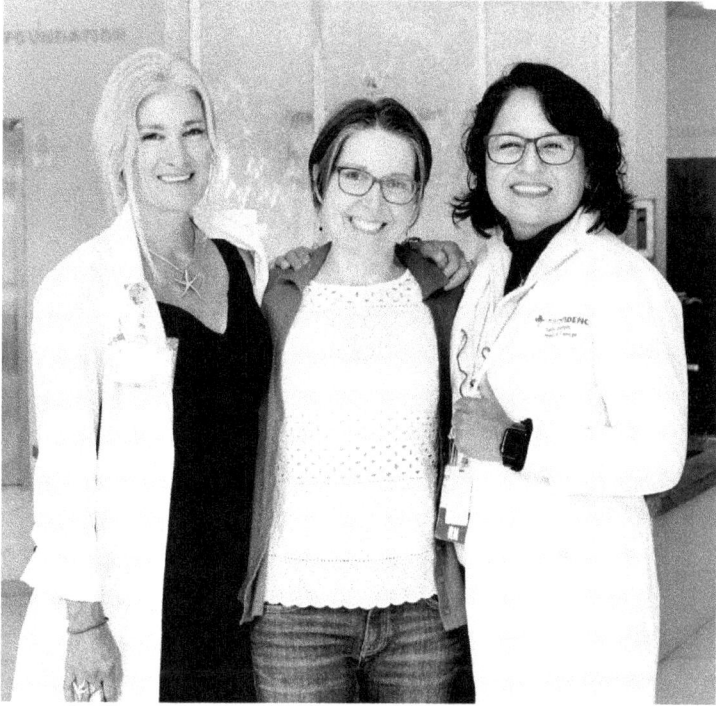
Rémy and Martha

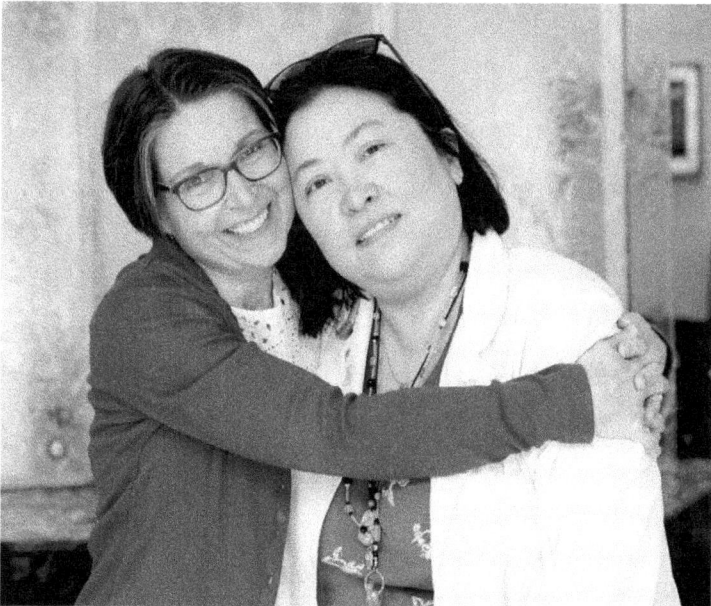
Radiation Nurse, Cindy

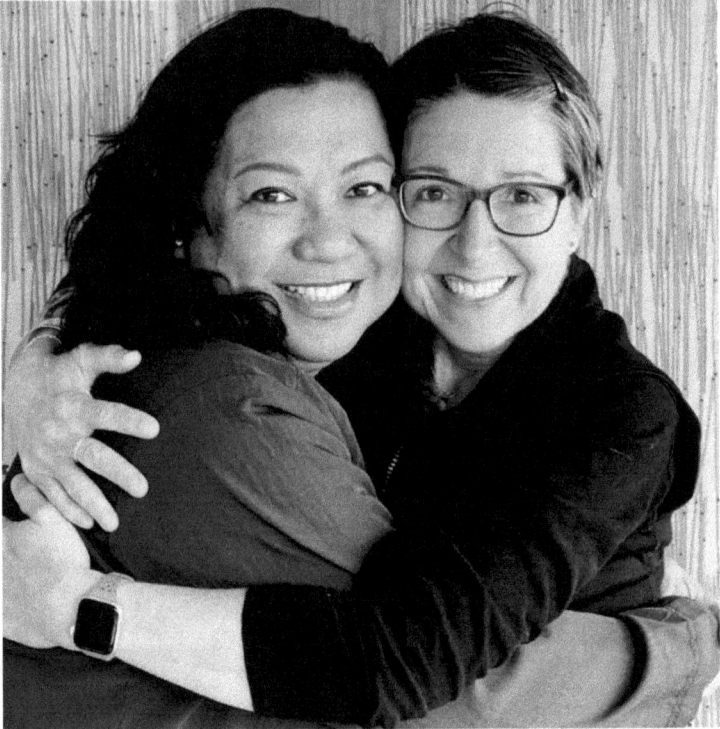

Infusion Nurse, Abby

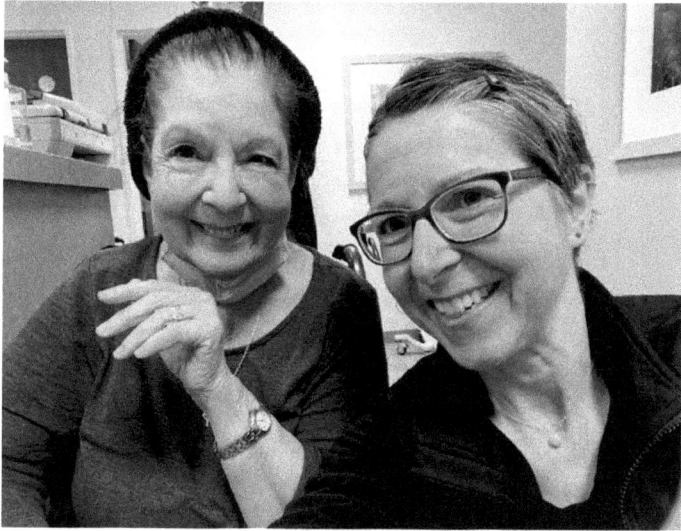

Vicky

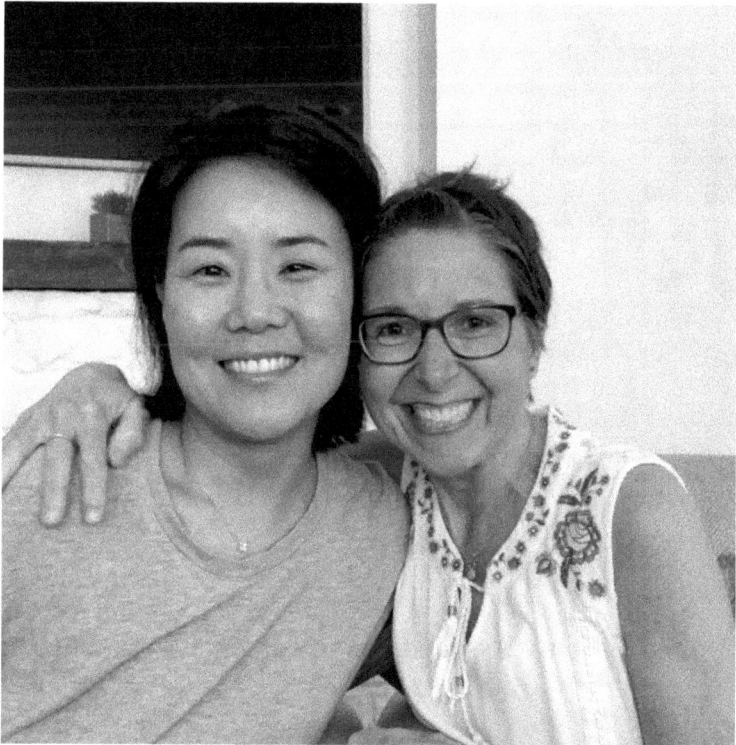

Suzy

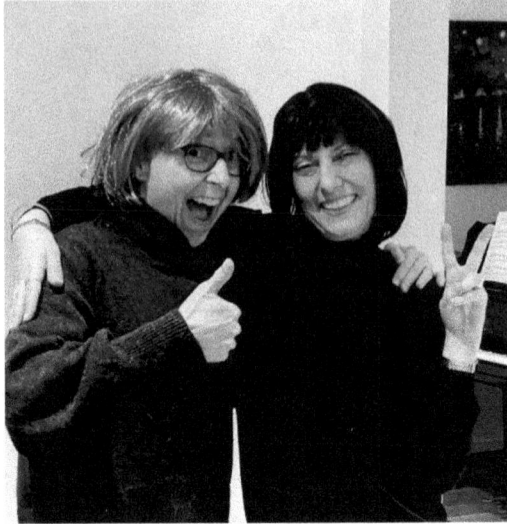

Traci

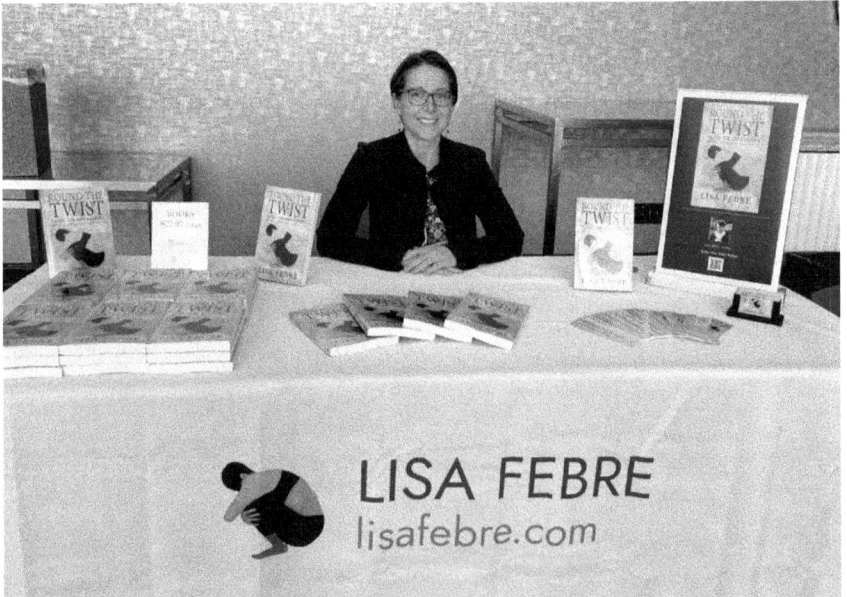

United Ostomy Associations of America Book Sale, August
2023

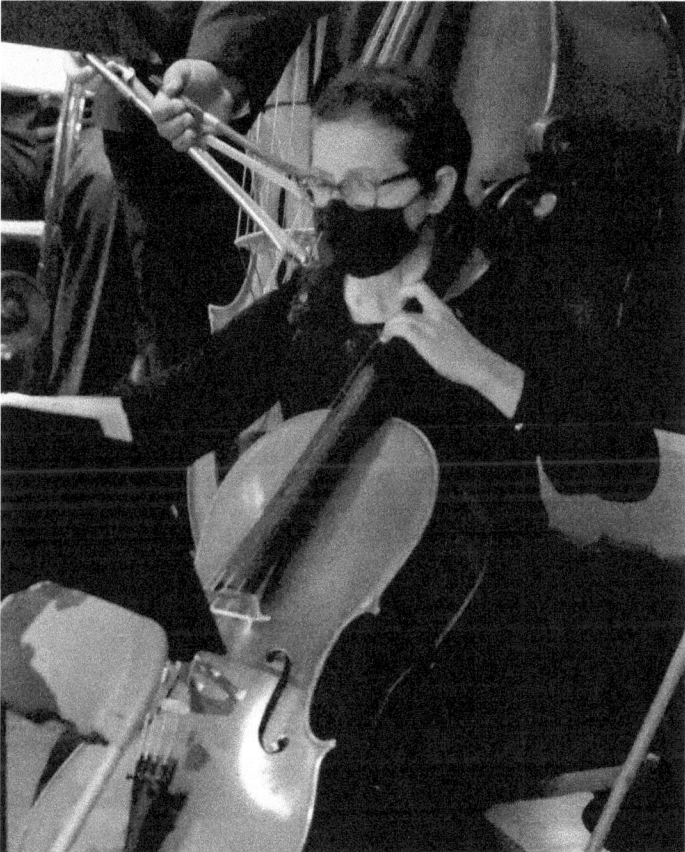

First concert after cancer

Celebrating One-Year Post Chemo

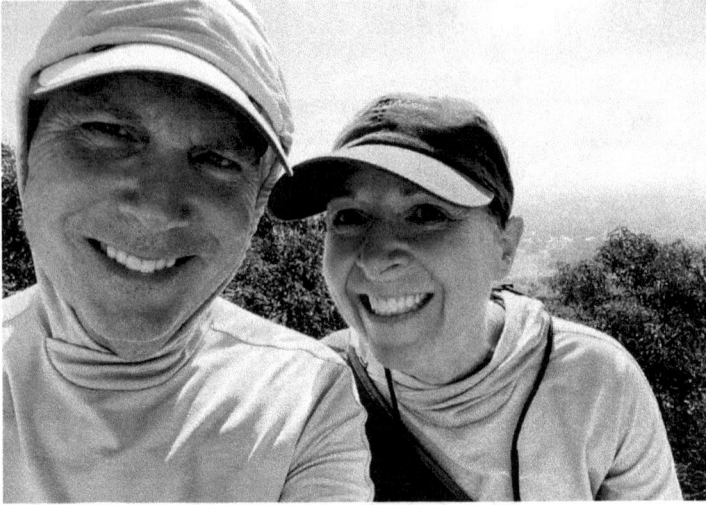

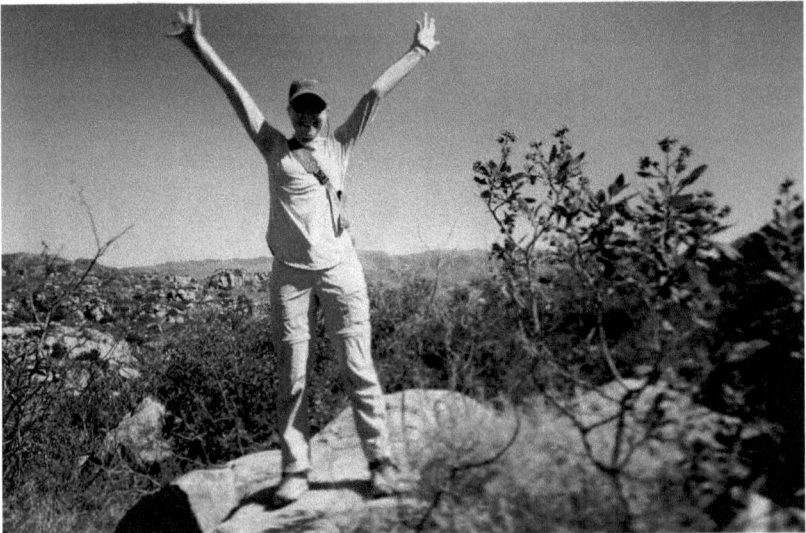

Message from the Author

Recovering from cancer and its treatments is not only about the physical toll. Our mental health can be greatly affected by the experience. There is no shame in needing support or professional help to get through the residual side-effects. When your doctor asks you, "How are you doing?" this is the time to be honest and let them know all the things you are going through. This includes your emotional struggles.

Just as it takes a team of oncologists to fight our cancer, we also need a team of professionals to battle our inner demons.

Find the help you need to get back to living your best life. You are not alone.

About the Author

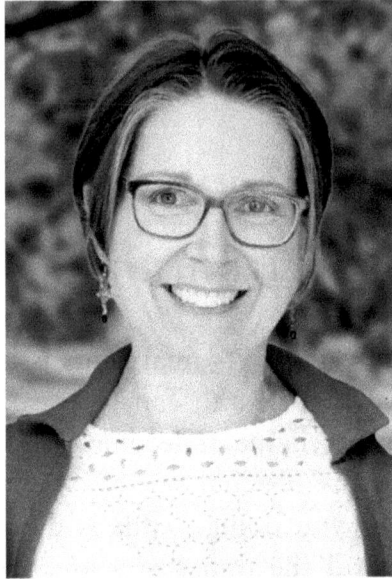

Lisa Febre spent the first three and a half decades of her life in a westward migration from New England to the Pacific Ocean. A musician since the age of 4, writing found her later in life when she published her first book, *"Round the Twist: Facing the Abdominable,"* at the age of 47.

Her diagnosis with colon cancer not only changed the trajectory of her life but also her career. Lisa loves the stage whether that is performing on cello or giving public presentations about her journey and how a positive attitude can greatly influence treatment outcomes. Lisa lives in Chatsworth, CA with her husband Louis, son Andrew, and rescue dogs Dusty and Luna.

Other Titles by Lisa Febre

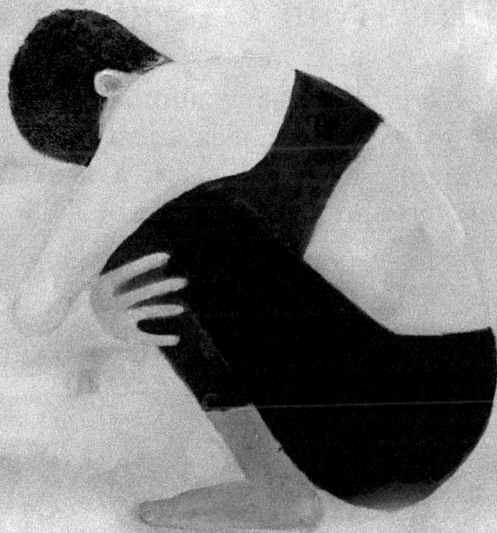

ROUND THE
TWIST
FACING THE ABDOMINABLE
Memoir of a Young Colon Cancer Survivor

LISA FEBRE

Note from Lisa Febre

Word-of-mouth is crucial for any author to succeed. If you enjoyed *Welcome to the Bright*, please leave a review online—anywhere you are able. Even if it's just a sentence or two, it would make all the difference and would be very much appreciated.

Thanks!
Lisa Febre

We hope you enjoyed reading this title from:

BLACK ROSE
writing™

Subscribe to our mailing list – *The Rosevine* – and receive **FREE** books, daily deals, and stay current with news about upcoming releases and our hottest authors.
Scan the QR code below to sign up.

Already a subscriber? Please accept a sincere thank you for being a fan of Black Rose Writing authors.

View other Black Rose Writing titles at
www.blackrosewriting.com/books and use promo code
PRINT to receive a **20% discount** when purchasing.